Amani Kacem
Rahma Benjazia
Zaineb Ouertani

Bronchial Dilatation:

Amani Kacem
Rahma Benjazia
Zaineb Ouertani

Bronchial Dilatation:

An Underestimated Respiratory Burden

ScienciaScripts

Imprint
Any brand names and product names mentioned in this book are subject to trademark, brand or patent protection and are trademarks or registered trademarks of their respective holders. The use of brand names, product names, common names, trade names, product descriptions etc. even without a particular marking in this work is in no way to be construed to mean that such names may be regarded as unrestricted in respect of trademark and brand protection legislation and could thus be used by anyone.

Cover image: www.ingimage.com

This book is a translation from the original published under ISBN 978-620-6-72744-6.

Publisher:
Sciencia Scripts
is a trademark of
Dodo Books Indian Ocean Ltd. and OmniScriptum S.R.L publishing group

120 High Road, East Finchley, London, N2 9ED, United Kingdom
Str. Armeneasca 28/1, office 1, Chisinau MD-2012, Republic of Moldova, Europe
Printed at: see last page
ISBN: 978-620-8-31145-2

TABLE OF CONTENTS

INTRODUCTION

Bronchial dilatation (BDD) or bronchiectasis was first described by Laennec as a chronic lung condition characterised by a permanent and irreversible increase in bronchial calibre (1). This disease is linked to destruction of the musculo-elastic and cartilaginous framework of the bronchus, affecting the portion between the 4th and 8th bronchial divisions(1). Clinical symptoms are dominated by chronic bronchorrhoea, which is the main symptom. symptoms and haemoptysis, which can be life-threatening(2). A thoracic CT scan is an essential diagnostic tool, enabling a distinction to be made between localised and diffuse bronchial dilatation. This distinction is important, as localised bronchial dilatation is usually the result of a localised cause (tumour, lymph node compression, foreign body), whereas diffuse bronchial dilatation has many aetiologies(3).Epidemiologically, there has been an upward trend in the prevalence of DDB in recent years, with significant social and health consequences. (4) The prevalence of DDB unrelated to cystic fibrosis is approximately 14 per 10,000.inhabitants in the United States (5) and has been on the rise since the 2000s, at a rate of approximately+8% per year (6.7) . As a result, there has been a resurgence of interest in this condition, which was once classed as an orphan disease, with an increase in the number of cases diagnosed. This is due to the wider availability of CT scans and their more frequent use, but also to greater awareness of the clinical picture. However, the disease continues to be under-diagnosed. This chronic respiratory disease has considerable morbidity and results in significant consumption of healthcare resources. It is therefore necessary to quantify the impact of DDB on quality of life and identify the patients most at risk. of unfavourable evolution. Scores developed specifically for this purpose can help clinicians in their work. Physiological and microbiological variables and the frequency of exacerbations are useful in the initial assessment and follow-up of patients with DDB. Taken together in the form of scores and combined with the extent of bronchiectasis on chest CT scan, these variables make it possible to anticipate hospital admissions and determine the vital prognosis of these patients(6). We believe that knowledge of the radio-clinical profile, the aetiologies of DDB and their evolutionary profile will enable better prevention of the disease and its possible complications. The clinical presentation and prognosis of the disease are heterogeneous, differing according to the profile of the patients and their origins, the clinical and radiological features and the aetiology of the disease.To our knowledge, there are no descriptive studies of the profile of DDB in the kairouan region.

The aim of our work is therefore to:

- To draw up a radio-clinical, aetiological and evolutionary profile of patients treated for diffuse bronchial dilatation in the Kairouan region.

- Research and analyse the factors influencing the frequency o f exacerbations in

DDB.

MATERIALS AND METHODS

1. TYPE OF STUDY :

This is a retrospective descriptive study of 100 patients with bronchial dilatation treated in the pneumo-allergology department at Ibn Al Jazzar Hospital in Kairouan, collected over a period of 10 years, from January 2010 to December 2020.

2. STUDY POPULATION :

2.1. TARGET POPULATION :

All patients diagnosed with bronchial dilatation between January 2010 and December 2020.

2.2. INCLUSION CRITERIA :

All patients treated for DDB were included. The diagnosis was made on the basis of suggestive clinical signs and confirmed by chest CT scan. Confirmation is provided by scans based on the presence of bronchi with a bronchial diameter/arterial diameter ratio > 1 or an absence of reduction in bronchial calibre with bronchial tubes less than 1cm from the pleura.

2.3. NON-INCLUSION CRITERIA :

Not all patients were included in the study: Whose diagnostic approach has not been finalised. Who do not have a chest CT scan.

2.4. EXCLUSION CRITERIA :

Traction DDB as part of fibrosing diffuse interstitial lung disease (DIP).

3. DATA COLLECTION :

Epidemiological, clinical and paraclinical data were collected, as well as data relating to the aetiological diagnosis, the impact of the disease, its management and its evolution. The epidemiological data collected includes age, sex and living environment. For each patient, smoking, ex-smoking or non-smoking status was recorded. Personal and family respiratory and extra-respiratory histories were sought and included: history of pulmonary tuberculosis, recurrent lung infections, severe respiratory infections in childhood, asthma, chronic obstructive pulmonary disease, lung cancer, systemic diseases, chronic IPD, infertility, radiotherapy, heart disease, diabetes and gastro-oesophageal reflux disease (GERD).

Regarding the circumstances of discovery, it was noted whether the discovery was fortuitous and the symptoms sought were cough, bronchorrhoea, haemoptysis, dyspnoea according to the mMRC scale, alteration in general condition, chest pain and fever.

On physical examination, pulmonary auscultation revealed crackles, sibilance and snoring, or was normal. We also looked for signs of chronic pulmonary heart disease, digital hippocratism and thoracic deformity (distension).

Abnormalities present on the chest X-ray, such as areolar images, tubular cleartes, cystic images, an air bronchogram with dilated bronchi, emphysema, sequellar images, pleurisy, cardiomegaly and atelectasis have been described.

On chest CT, the presence of cylindrical, cystic and varicose lesions, mixed cylindrical and cystic lesions, bronchial micronodules, ventilatory disorders, mediastinal adenopathy and situs inversus were noted.

The distribution of lesions was also specified.

The results of the following additional tests were specified: blood count (CBC), C reactive protein (CRP) and creatinine levels. Microbiological status was recorded using data from the results of the sputum cytobacteriological examination (SCE) and the bacteriological examination of the bronchial aspirate (BAL).

We recorded the results of functional respiratory investigations (FRI) by spirometry and specified the presence of obstructive ventilatory disorder (OVD), restrictive ventilatory disorder (RVD), mixed ventilatory disorder, forced expiratory volume in one second (FEV1), forced vital capacity (FVC), Tiffeneau ratio (TR), Body Mass Index (BMI) and arterial blood gas (ABG). The results of the 6-minute walk test, transthoracic echocardiography (TTE) and electrocardiogram (ECG) were collected.

The aetiologies of DDB were specified, such as idiopathic DDB, post-tuberculosis DDB, DDB secondary to repeated infections, cystic fibrosis, kartagener's syndrome and others.

We specified the medical and surgical therapeutic management during hospitalisation and in the stable state. We noted the use of beta 2 mimetics, inhaled corticoids, mucolytics, long-term macrolides, antibiotics and their duration, and physiotherapy.

We also noted patients using long-term oxygen therapy (LTO) and of

non-invasive ventilation (NIV) at home.

Diagnosis of severity was made using the FACED and bronchiectasis severity index (BSI) scores. Factors predictive of frequent exacerbations (>2) were determined.

We recorded data on the clinical course, such as the number of hospital admissions and complications such as haemoptysis, chronic respiratory failure (CRF) and death.

4. DEFINITIONS OF VARIABLES

A. SMOKING STATUS :

-Smoker: any patient who has smoked one cigarette a day or more for at least one year. Non-smoker: any patient who has smoked less than one cigarette a day and/or less than one year.
-Ex-smoker: any patient who has stopped smoking for more than one year.

B. THORACIC IMAGING DATA :

- **Chest X-ray :**

The images that can be seen are thick-walled, irregular, tubular cleartes, areolar images of variable size, cystic images with or without a fluid level, "immersion finger", "v", "y" or "cluster" opacities and an aeric bronchogram made up of dilated bronchi.

- **Chest CT :**

Diffuse DDB is the term used to describe bronchial dilatation affecting several lobes of a single lung. or both lungs, and localized DDB when it affects only one lobe of the lung.
According to the REID classification (7), a distinction is made between :

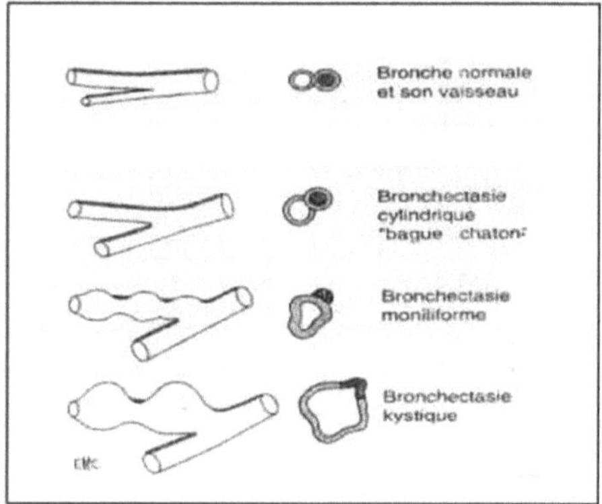

Classification de Reid

Figure 1: Reid classification

► Regular expansion :

Cylindrical bronchiectasis: the bronchi appear as tubes uniformly dilated along their lumens and visible close to the pleura (10mm from the parietal pleura, in contact with the mediastinal pleura).

► Varicose or moniliform :

The bronchial tubes resemble the dilatation of varicose veins. The dilatation is irregular and distal, with several stenoses appearing in a string.

► Sacciform or cystic :

Located at the end of the bronchi, leading to obstruction of the bronchioles downstream, the bronchi appear bloated with no recognisable structure and take on an ampullary or cystic appearance.

C. SEVERITY DIAGNOSIS :

► THE FACED SCORE

The FACED score is a score established to assess the severity of patients with non-mucoviscidosis bronchiectasis. Seven variables are taken into account: FEV1; the presence or absence of Pseudomonas oruginosa colonisation; the MMRC dyspnoea score; age; and the number of lobes affected on chest X-ray (8).

D. EXACERBATIONS :

An exacerbation is defined by the presence of at least three of the following symptoms for at least 48 hours (cough, increased sputum volume, sputum purulence, dyspnoea, haemoptysis, fatigue or malaise)(9)

The combination of two exacerbations or one hospitalisation per year is the definition of a frequent exacerbator, which has the best predictive value for mortality, regardless of the initial severity of the bronchiectasis(10).

5. PROGRESS OF THE STUDY :

The pre-established medical questionnaire was completed by the investigator for patients with bronchial dilatation confirmed by a thoracic CT scan and who were being followed in the pulmonology department.

5. STATISTICAL ANALYSIS :

The data were entered and analysed using SPSS version 22.0 software. The analysis A descriptive and an analytical study were carried out.Qualitative variables were presented as percentages and quantitative variables as means or median (extreme) if their distribution did not follow a normal distribution. Qualitative variables were compared using Pearson's x2 test or Fisher's exact test according to the theoretical number of participants. Quantitative variables were compared using Student's t-test. The difference between two variables was considered significant if $p<0.05$.

A uni-variate study was carried out, in which each variable was studied independently of the others.

Those associated with a $p \leq 0.2$ were then entered into a stepwise linear descending regression model to identify those that were independently associated with more frequent exacerbations. The design threshold was set at 5%.

6. KEYWORDS AND SEARCH ENGINE

The results of our work were compared with data from recent literature and with the results of certain national and international series.

The bibliographical search was carried out using the main scientific search engines:

- www.Pubmed.com
- www.Sciencedirect.com

7. ETHICAL CONSIDERATIONS :

Certain ethical aspects were taken into consideration when carrying out this study:

• Confidentiality of data collected ;
• Respect for professional secrecy ;

We declare that there is no conflict of interest in this work.

RESULTS

I. EPIDEMIOLOGICAL DATA :

During the study period, 100 patients were enrolled.

1. BREAKDOWN BY AGE AND GENDER:

The mean age of patients in our study was 57.97 years, with extremes ranging from 17 to 90 years old.There was a predominance of women, with 55 women (55%) and 45 men (45%). The sex ratio (male/female) was 0.81. The distribution by gender and age group showed :

•A peak in frequency in the over-65 age group.

• A predominance of men in the under-25 a g e group. Above that age women predominate.

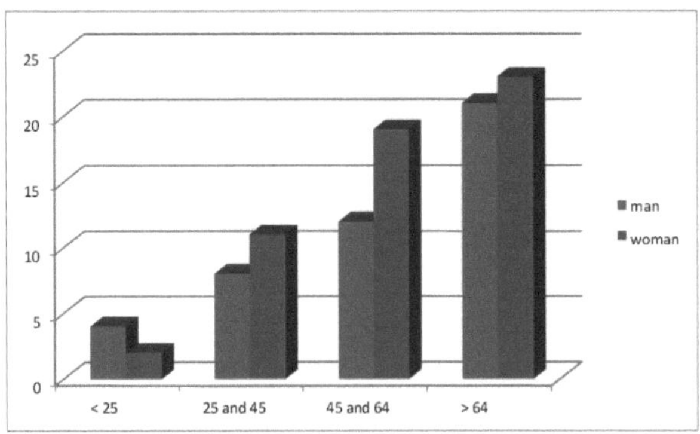

Figure 2: Distribution of patients by age group and sex

2. BREAKDOWN BY GEOGRAPHICAL ORIGIN :

Sixty-nine of our patients (69%) were of rural origin, and 31 patients were of rural origin. Urban (31%).

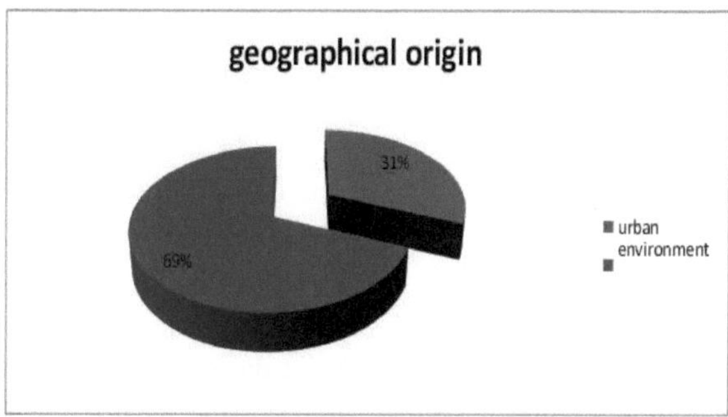

Figure 3: Breakdown of patients by geographical origin

3. SMOKING AND PATHOLOGICAL ANTECEDENTS:

► **Smoking :**

Of the 100 patients, 37 were smokers or ex-smokers. The number of pack-years (PY) varied between 5 and 120 PY, with an average of 48.4 PY.

Table I: Distribution of patients according to smoking habits

Toxic History	Number of patients	Average consumption in P/A
Active smoking	28	50
Ex-smoker	9	43
No smoking	63	-

► **History:**

o **Respiratory history :**

The patient's medical history was marked by a predominance of respiratory pathologies. The results are shown in Table II :

Table II: Distribution of patients according to pathological history

Pathological history	Number of patients n	Percentage
Pulmonary tuberculosis	40	40%
Repeated respiratory infections	21	21%
COPD	20	20%
Asthma	12	12%
Respiratory infections in childhood	9	9%
Bronchial tumour	4	4%
COPD: obstructive pulmonary disease		

- **Non-respiratory history:**

Extra pulmonary antecedents were dominated by cardiovascular pathologies, with 12% of patients reporting heart disease and 10% diabetes. There has also been one case of adrenal insufficiency, one case of hypothyroidism, one case of psoriasis and one case of chronic sinusitis.

II. DATA CLINICAL:

1. CIRCUMSTANCES OF DISCOVERY :

All patients included in our study were symptomatic at the time of the first consultation. The functional signs found are dominated by bronchorrhoea and cough. Table III summarises the various tell-tale signs.

Table III: Distribution of patients according to clinical signs

Telltale signs	Number of patients n	Percentage
Productive cough (bronchorrhoea)	80	80%
Dyspnoea	61	61%
Haemoptysis	34	34%
Impaired general condition	26	26%
Chest pain	24	24%
Fever	20	20%

2. Physical examination :

○ **Pleuropulmonary examination :**

At the time of data collection, pleural and pulmonary examinations were normal in 06 patients (6%.Polypnoea with a respiratory rate of between 20 cycles per minute and 38 cycles per minute was noted in 47 patients (47%). Signs of struggle such as intercostal and supra-sternal pulling, paradoxical abdominal breathing, contraction of the accessory respiratory muscles and pursed-lip breathing were found in 31 patients (31%). Pulmonary auscultation showed a predominance of snoring sounds in 51.9% of patients. Table IV summarises the results of pulmonary auscultation.

Table IV: Signs observed during pulmonary auscultation

Auscultation	Number of patients n	Percentage
Crepitating rales	70	70%
Rumbles	40	40%
Sibilant rales	25	25%

❖ Extra pulmonary examination :

In addition to the pleuropulmonary examination, the physical examination can be used to look for signs in favour of an aetiology (congenital malformation) or signs testifying to the repercussions of DDB (signs of chronic pulmonary heart disease (CPC), digital hippocratism, thoracic deformity).

Table V: Physical signs noted in patients

Physical sign	Number of patients n	Percentage
Digital hippocratism	36	36%
Signs of insufficiency right heart	16	16%
Chest deformity (distension)	5	5%

III. PARA-CLINICAL DATA :

1. Examination radiology:

► **Chest X-ray :**

All patients had a frontal chest X-ray. Chest X-ray abnormalities and their distribution were recorded. The most frequently observed radiological aspect in the population studied was a bronchial syndrome with areolar images in 55% of cases. The lesions were bilateral in 70% of cases and unilateral in 30%. The radiological abnormalities visible on the X-rays are shown in Table VI.

Table VI: Chest X-ray abnormalities

Radiological abnormality	Number of patients n	Percentage
areolar image	55	55%
Cystic images	42	42%
Air bronchogram with dilated bronchi	39	39%
Emphysema/thoracic distension	23	23%
After-effect images	21	21%
Alveolar opacity	18	18%
Atelectasis	11	11%
Tubal clarity	8	8%
Cardiomegaly	7	7%
Pleuresis	3	3%

Figures 4, 5, 6 and 7 illustrate some of the radiological aspects observed in our patients.

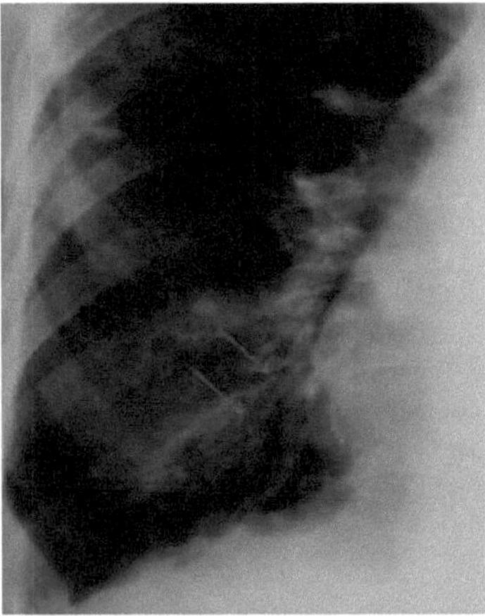

Figure 4: chest X-ray showing tubulated <rail> images.

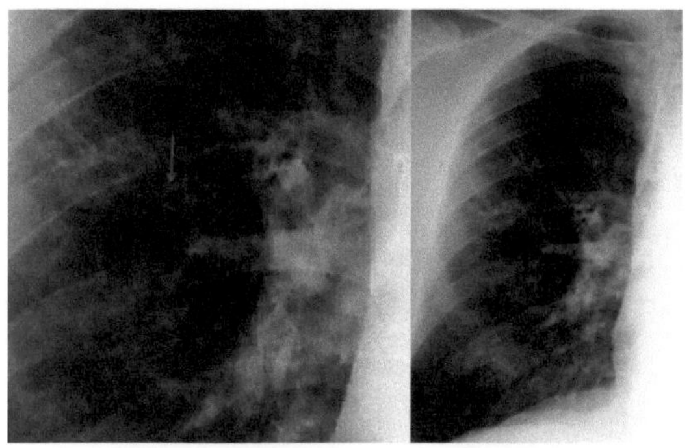

Figure 5: Chest X-ray showing "ring" images

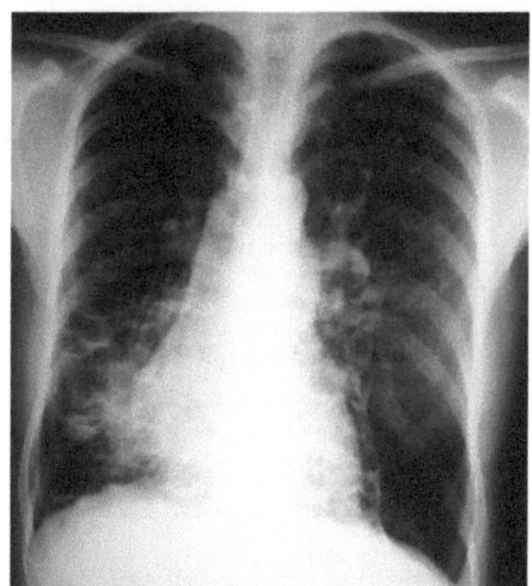

Figure 6: Chest X-ray showing cystic images

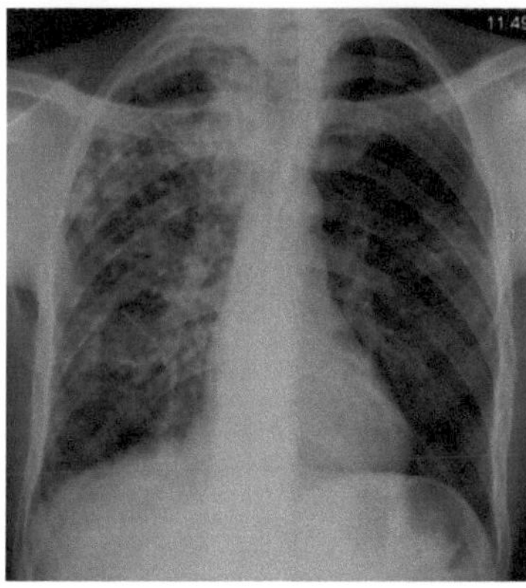

Figure 7: Chest X-ray showing V-shaped images

► Chest computed tomography :

The diagnosis of DDB was based on high-resolution chest CT. Confirmation of the diagnosis of DDB was obtained in 100% of cases by thoracic CT scan.

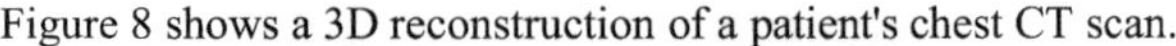
Figure 8 shows a 3D reconstruction of a patient's chest CT scan.

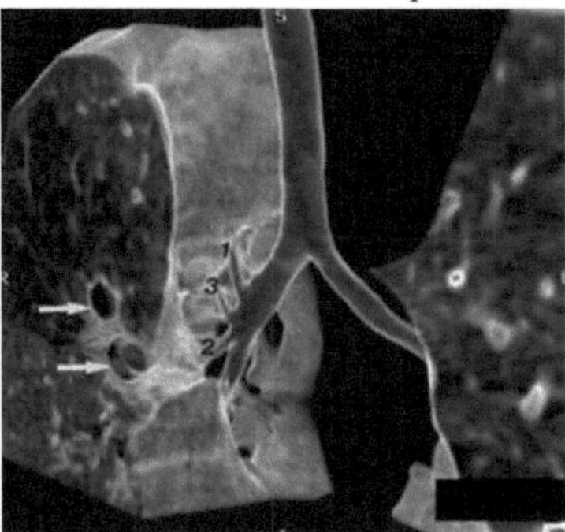

Figure 8: 3D reconstruction of a chest CT scan

► Type of lesions :

The types of scannographic lesions found are shown in Table VIII.

Table VII: Types of abnormalities present on thoracic CT scan

CT appearance	Number of patients n	Percentage
Cylindrical lesions	75	75%
Cystic lesions	52	52%
Varicose lesions	19	19%
Mixed cylindrical lesions and cystic	32	32%
Bronchial micronodules	46	46%
Ventilatory disorders (atelectasis)	22	22%
Mediastinal adenopathy	16	16%
Situs inversus	3	3%

Figures 9, 10 and 11 show the different scans observed.

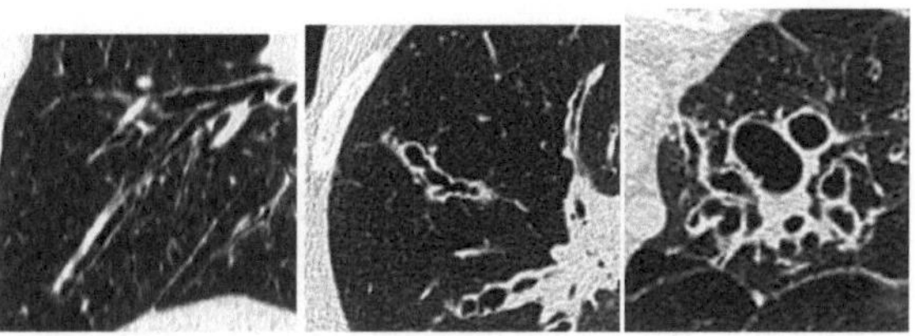

Figure 9Figure 10Figure 11

Figure 9: shows a cylindrical DDB (parallel walls of the bronchi)

Figure 10: shows varicose DDB with a succession of narrowings and dilations

Figure 11: shows a cystic DDB with frank dilatation and the presence of hydroaerobic levels.

► Scope and registered office :

The DDBs were diffuse in 67% of cases and localised in 33%. Diffuse DDB refers to bronchial dilatation affecting several lobes of one or both lungs. These lesions were bilateral in 88% of cases and unilateral in 22%.

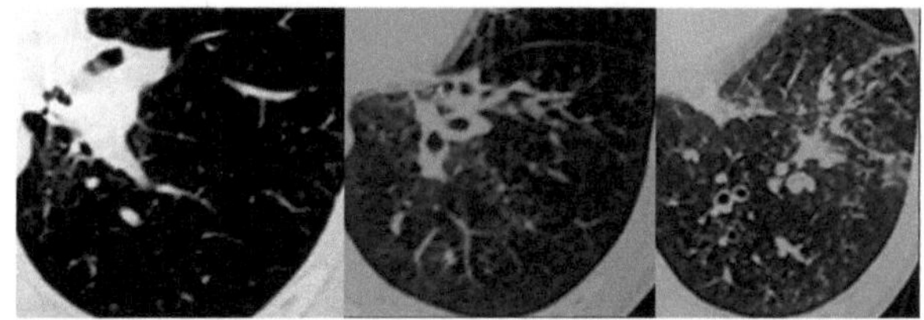

Figure 12: Localized DDB due to inhalation of a foreign body

2. BIOLOGICAL DATA :

- The mean leucocyte count was 8969.9/mm^3 with extremes ranging from 3100/mm^3 to 20000/mm^3).

- Hyperleukocytosis (white blood cells(WBC) 2: 12000/mm3) was noted in 18 patients.

(18%) with a predominance of neutrophils (PNN) in 10% of cases.

- Leukopenia (WBC <4000/mm^3) was noted in 2 patients (2%).
- Haemoglobinemia of less than 10g/dl was noted in 11 patients (11%).

-The mean platelet count was 277670/mm^3 [110,000/mm^3 to 616,000/mm^3].

- Thrombocytopenia of less than 150,000/mm^3 was noted in 6 patients (6%) and thrombocytosis of more than 450,000/mm^3 was found in 7 patients (7%).

- All our patients had had a CRP test, with elevated CRP (>5) in 30% of cases.
- 3 patients developed renal failure.

3. Microbiological status :

Microbiological status was recorded using data from ECBC and BAL examinations, which were performed in 19 patients. We isolated the germ in 63% of cases. The germs found were: Streptococcus pneumoniae in 4 cases, Pseudomonas aeruginosa in 5 cases, Candidas albicans in 2 cases and Staphylococcus aureus in 1 case. The results are shown in Figure 13.

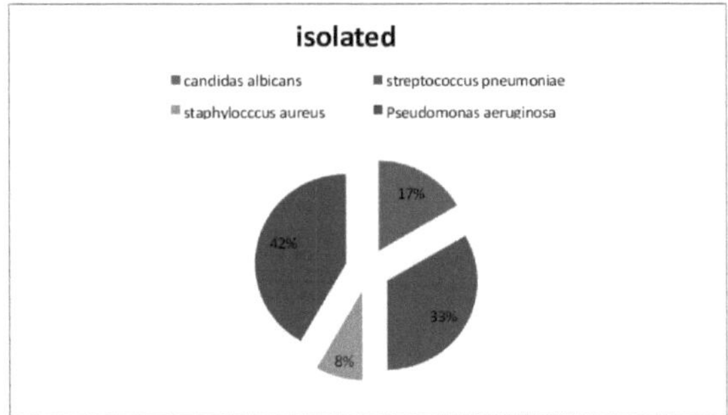

Figure 13: Germs isolated in the cytobacteriological examination of sputum

4. Bronchial fibroscopy :

Six of our patients underwent bronchial fibroscopy, which showed a normal appearance in 3 patients (50%), an inflammatory appearance in 2 patients, and bleeding in one patient. In addition, no endobronchial lesions were found, in particular a bud. stenosis or extrinsic compression.

IV. ETIOLOGICAL DIAGNOSIS :

1. ETIOLOGICAL ASSESSMENT :

The aetiological work-up is based essentially on taking the main personal and family histories and carrying out a series of additional tests to identify the main aetiologies.

1.1. History :

We noted a personal history of pulmonary tuberculosis (40%), a family history of DDB (4%) and severe respiratory infections in childhood (9%).

1.2. Chest CT :

Chest CT confirmed the diagnosis of bronchial dilatation, but also revealed associated abnormalities such as signs suggestive of pulmonary tuberculosis sequelae in 10 patients (10%), situs inversus in 3 cases, mediastinal adenopathy in 16% of cases, and thus contributed to the aetiological diagnosis in 29% of cases.

1.3. Bronchial fibroscopy :

Bronchial fibroscopy is an essential examination in the aetiological assessment, particularly in the case of localised DDB, in order to search for a foreign body, an endobronchial lesion or extrinsic compression. None of these anomalies were noted in our study.

1.4. Tuberculosis work-up :

Testing for BK in sputum revealed 4 cases of active tuberculosis. An intradermal tuberculin test (IDR) was carried out in 20 cases, with negative results. BK was tested in bronchial aspirates, which were also negative.

1.5. Others :

The anti-SCL 70 antibody test was positive in 1 case and the diagnosis of scleroderma was accepted.Testing for anti-nuclear antibodies (ANA) was not systematic in all patients, and no positive results were reported. There have been cases of rheumatoid arthritis in which rheumatoid factor has been measured. Weighted immunoglobulin (Ig) assays were carried out in only 5 patients, and concluded in IgG deficiency in one.

2. ETIOLOGIES :

An aetiology was selected in 68 cases, i.e. 68%. We noted a predominance of post-tuberculous DDB in 40 cases, followed by DDB secondary to repeated infections in 14 cases. Post-radiation DDB in 4 cases and kartagener's syndrome in 3 cases. Figure 14 summarises the main aetiologies found in our series.

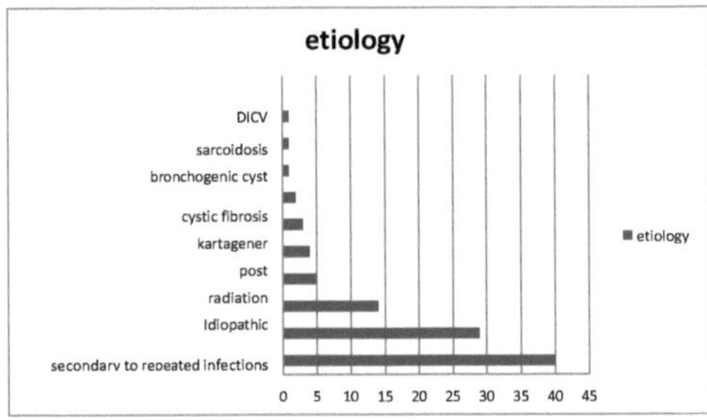

Figure 14: The main causes of DDB

Figures 15, 16, 17 and 18 illustrate radiological aspects pointing to the etiology of DDB.

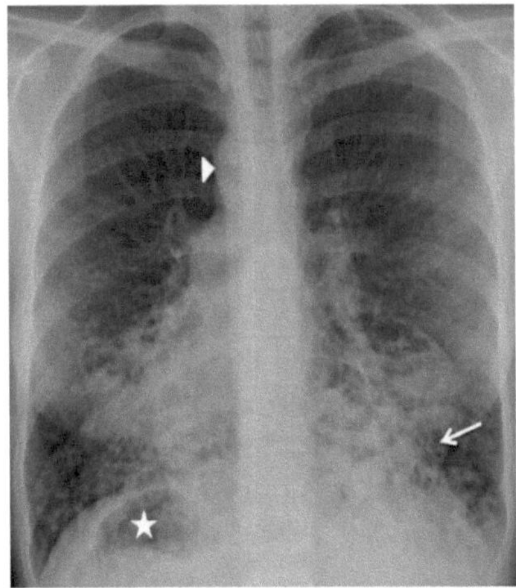

Figure 15: Chest X-ray showing kartagener's syndrome

•

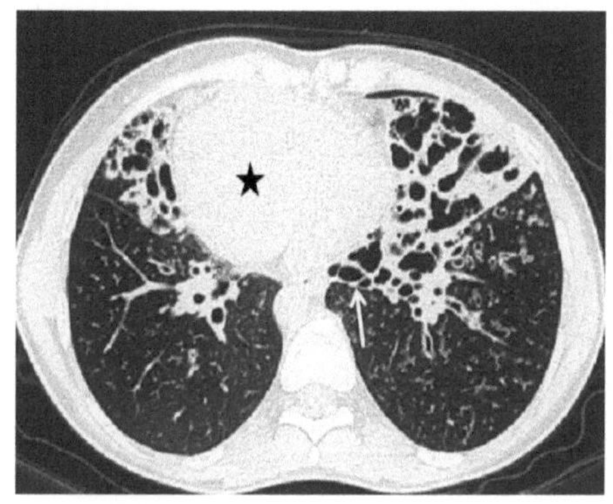

Figure 16: a chest scan showing kartagener's syndrome

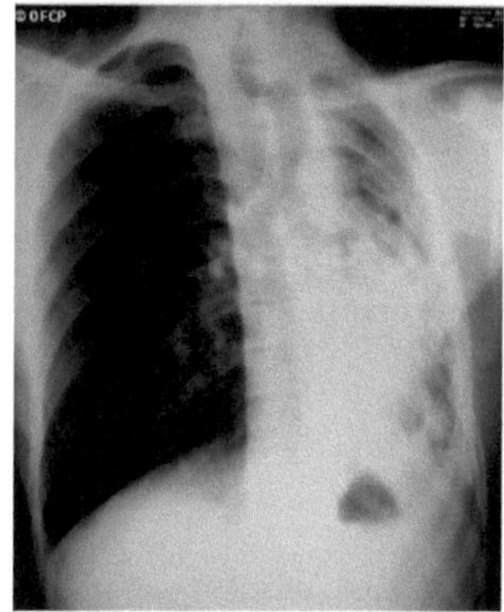

Figure 17: Chest X-ray showing post-tuberculous DDB

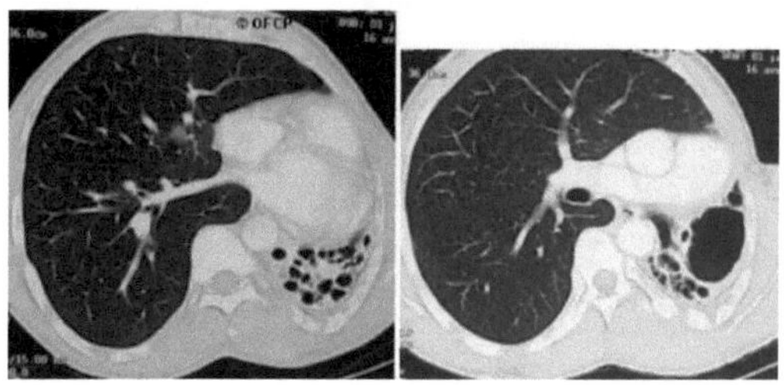

Figure 18: Chest CT scan showing post-tuberculous DDB

V. IMPACT ASSESSMENT :

1. FUNCTIONAL RESPIRATORY INVESTIGATIONS (FRI) :

1.1. Spirometry :

Spirometry was performed in 55 patients (55%), showing an obstructive syndrome in 22 patients, a restrictive tendency in 6 cases and a mixed syndrome in 15 patients.

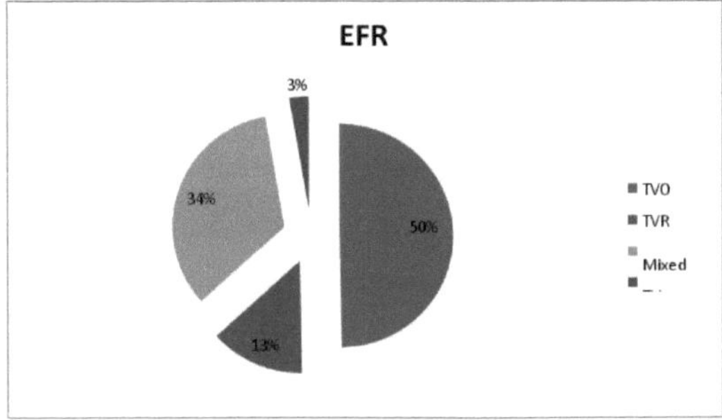

Figure 19: Functional abnormalities detected by spirometry in our patients

1.2. Arterial blood gas :

Arterial blood gas analysis was performed on admission in 89 patients. It showed hypoxaemia (PaO_2<60) in 27 patients. Ten patients were hypercapnic ($PaCO_2$ 2: 45 mm Hg) and 52 patients had correct blood gases.

The various gasometric data are shown in Table 8.

Table VIII: Arterial blood gas data

Parameter	Minimum	Maximum	Median
HCO3-	15	45	26
PaO2	35	131	68
PCO2	20	79	40
SaO2	70	99	90

HCO3-: bicarbonate ions, Pao2: arterial oxygen pressure, PCO2: arterial oxygen pressure.

arterial carbon dioxide, SaO2: Pulse Oxygen Saturation

1.3. 6-minute walk test :

The 6-minute walk test was performed in 10 patients (10%). Two patients (20%) had a severe limitation with a walking distance of less than 150 metres. Moderate limitation was found in 5 patients (50%) and no functional limitation of the walking perimeter was found in 3 patients (30%).

2. CARDIAC ULTRASOUND :

Cardiac echocardiography was performed in 60 patients, showing PH in 16 patients with an estimated mean systolic pulmonary artery pressure (PAPs) of 42.5.

VI. THERAPEUTIC MANAGEMENT :

1. MEDICAL TREATMENT :

1.1 ANTIBIOTIC THERAPY :

During hospitalisation, 96 patients were treated with probabilistic antibiotics.The choice of antibiotic family was based on clinical orientation,radiological and bacteriological. Amoxicillin-clavulanic acid, used in 80% of cases, was the drug most commonly used as monotherapy.In dual therapy, the combinations used were 3rd generation cephalosporin (C3G) + fluoroquinolones or C3G + aminoglycosides.The average duration of antibiotic treatment was 7 days [1 day - 26 days].

1.2KINESITHERAPY :

Respiratory physiotherapy was performed in 70 patients (70%).

1.3OTHER THERAPIES :

Patients received other therapies depending on the severity of the clinical signs. 35% of patients received intravenous corticosteroids. Other therapeutic measures have been put in place to improve patients' quality of life, apart from superinfections and hospitalisation. These are summarised in the table below.

Table IX: Therapeutic measures in the stable state

Therapeutic measure	percentage
inhaled corticosteroids	88%
beta2-mimetics	85%
Mucolytics	30%

Smoking cessation, dental care, flu and pneumococcal vaccinations have all been recommended. was indicated in 80% of patients.

2.SURGICAL TREATMENT :

Surgery was indicated in 4 patients. In these patients, the indication for surgery was recurrent lower respiratory infections or threatening haemoptysis. Two patients underwent right lower lobe lobectomy, 1 middle lobe lobectomy and 1 left upper lobe lobectomy.

VII. EVOLUTION AND COMPLICATIONS :

► **Chronic respiratory failure (CRF) :**

Chronic respiratory failure was found in 30 cases requiring home oxygen, and 15 cases required long-term non-invasive ventilation (NIV).

► **Haemoptysis :**

In our series, 7 cases of haemoptysis were reported, 4 of which required embolisation and 3 progressed well with symptomatic treatment.

► **Exacerbations requiring hospitalisation :**

46% of patients in our series had an average of >2 hospitalisations per year, with 11 patients admitted to the intensive care unit. Emergency NIV was used in 23% of cases and 6 patients were intubated.

VIII. SEVERITY DIAGNOSIS :

1. SEVERITY SCORES :

According to the FACED score, the risk of mortality at 5 years was high in 12% of cases, moderate (in 20%) and low (in 68%). According to the bronchiectasis severity index (BSI) score, the risk of mortality and hospitalisation was high in 71% of cases and moderate in 26%.

IX ANALYTICAL PART

1. UNIVARIATE ANALYSIS

In our study, eight factors were identified as having a significant influence on the frequent exacerbations (>2 per year). In terms of antecedents, tuberculosis (p=0.002) was noted as a predictive factor.more frequent exacerbations.There was no significant difference between patients with a history of COPD (p=0.91) or heart disease (p=0.131). Among the clinical signs, the presence of dyspnoea as a revealing sign (p=0.003) and hypoxaemia (p=0.003) were associated with a higher number of exacerbations.We also noted that the presence of PAH on cardiac ultrasound (p=0.048) and the presence of respiratory failure (p=0.001) correlated with more frequent exacerbations.The presence of pseudomonas aeroginosa (p=0.019) also influenced the frequency of exacerbations.Respiratory function tests showed that the presence of an OVT (p=0.048) was also predictive of exacerbation. On thoracic CT, the diffuse distribution of lesions (p=0.053) is associated with a risk of exacerbations.

Table X: univariate analysis of factors predictive of exacerbations

Exacerbations P OR , IC,95%

	<2	>=2		
Age <65	25 (46,3%)	29	0,240	
>=65 years	16 (43,8%)	(53,7%)		
		30		
		(65,2%)		
Tobacco no	24 (40%)	36 (60%)	0,802	
yes	17 (42,5%)	23		
		(57,5%)		
Previous TBC			0,002	0,264 [0,113,
no	17 (28,3%)	43		0,614]
yes	24 (60%)	(71,7%)		
		16 (40%)		
History of COPD			0,91	
no	33 (41,3%)	47		
yes	16 (40%)	(58,8%)		
		4 (60%)		
History of heart disease				
no	39 (44,3%)	49	0,131	
yes	2 (16,7%)	(55,7%)		
		10		
		(83,3%)		
Dyspnoea no	23 (59%)	16 (41%)	0,003	3,434
yes	18 (29,5%)	43		[1,479,7,975]
		(70,5%)		
Digital hippocratism			0,241	
no	29 (45,3%)	35		
yes	12 (33,3%)	(54,7%)		
		24		
		(66,7%)		
Hypoxemia			0,003	3,674

no	31 (53,4%)	27		[1,527, 8,838]
yes	10 (23,8%)	(46,6%)		
		32		
		(76,2%)		
Signs of insufficiency			0,946	
right heart				
no	37 (41,1%)	53		
yes	4 (40%)	(58,9%)		
		6 (60%)		
Signs of PH			0,048	3,580
no	38 (45,2%)	46		[0,950, 13,493]
yes	3 (18,8%)	(54,8%)		
		13		
		(81,3%)		
Respiratory failure			0,001	14,884
no	40 (48,2%)	43		[1,886 , 117,439]
yes	1(5,9%)	(51,8%)		
		16		
		(94,1%)		
Presence of Pseudomonas			0,019	0,568
aerogenosa in sputum				[0,477, 0,677]
no	41 (43,2%)	54		
yes	0	(56,8%)		
		5 (100%)		
Thrombocytosis			0,917	
no	38 (40,9%)	55		
yes	3 (42,9%)	(59,1%)		
		4 (57,1%)		
TVO			0,048	2,914
no	36 (46,2%)	42		[0,978 , 8,685]
yes	5 (22,7%)	(53,8%)		
		17		
		(77,3%)		
Distribution of lesions			0,053	2,296
Diffuse	18 (54,5%)	15		[0,980 , 5,375]
Localised	23 (34,3%)	(45,5%)		
		44		
		(65,7%)		
Situs inversus			0,384	
no	41 (42,3%)	56		
yes	0	(57,7%)		
		3 (100%)		

TBC: tuberculosis, COPD: obstructive pulmonary disease, PH: pulmonary hypertension, OVD: obstructive ventilatory disorder

2. MULTIVARIATE ANALYSIS

Multivariate analysis showed that the presence of pseudomonas aeruginosa was a significant independent factor in frequent exaerbations.

Table XI: Multivariate analysis of factors predictive of exacerbations

	variableORa; 95% CI	P
The presence of pseudomonas	0,348 [0,127	0,039

DISCUSSION

Bronchial dilatation (BDD) is defined as a permanent and irreversible increase in the calibre of the bronchial tubes with impaired function(11).The pathophysiological mechanisms involved in the genesis of the disease and its perpetuation involve infectious, mechanical, environmental, toxic and host-related factors(12).Their prevalence is currently on the increase, probably due to greater use of thoracic CT scans. In fact, the diagnosis is radiological and the reference method is the thoracic CT scan(13).To date, epidemiological data on the prevalence of DDB and its presentation are not available. clinical trials are rare due to the lack of studies on this subject(14).Since DDB can be the cause of significant morbidity, it is important to know how to recognise it and how to diagnose it aetiologically(15).Our study is a retrospective descriptive study spread over 10 years and including all 100 patients. It aims to draw up a clinical, aetiological and prognostic profile of patients with DDB through the analysis of 100 observations collected over 10 years from 2010 to 2020.

I. STRENGTHS AND LIMITATIONS OF THE STUDY :

The main limitations of this study are the small sample size. A larger number of patients could have refined our results. However, although our study is smaller in number, it is more powerful because it is a study spread over a relatively long period of 10 years (from 2010 to 2020), which allows for good follow-up.In addition, the patients selected belonged to the same department and the adapted diagnostic approach and management were similar, which enabled a better assessment of the work methodology.As far as we know, this is the first study on this subject in the Kairouan region. Nevertheless, to compensate for these limitations, we would like to point out that inaccurate files have been excluded from the study.

II. DISCUSSION OF THE RESULTS

1.D EPIDEMIOLOGICAL DATA :

1.1.Age and gender :

DDB is an age-related disease.(16) A marked increase in prevalence, particularly of severe disease, is observed in the elderly(17).In our population, the average age was 57.97, and the majority was made up of women (55%), with a sex ratio of 0.81. Our population is similar to that of the Tunisian studies by Abdmouleh (18), Bejarand Trigui (20).The first is a retrospective study of 110 patients, with an average age of 60 years, while the second by Bejar (19) is a retrospective study of 85 patients, with an average age of 60.63 years. In his retrospective study including 50 patients, Trigui found an average age of 57.49. Worldwide, the age varies from country to country; in the UK it is around 52 (21), In Spain, the average age was 68.3 years (22).The decreased swallowing reflexes and increased prevalence of

GERD in the elderly may contribute to the development of DDB due to subclinical microaspiration including the nasopharyngeal microbiota (23). The elderly have a more severe disease and an atypical presentation with poorer outcomes than younger cohorts. (24)

1.2.Smoking and history :

In our series, smoking was reported in 37% of cases. A study carried out in Algeria (25) reported smoking in only 17% of cases. Boucher (26) has noted the effect of tobacco exposure on impaired mucociliary function. Smoking is also linked to a decline in respiratory function. It is also an independent risk factor for mortality from COPD(27). A new trend, the E cigarette or electronic cigarette, has been strongly suspected to have led to DDB according to a recent study carried out in California by Forest Ray(28) The most frequently reported respiratory histories in our series were tuberculosis (40%), recurrent respiratory infections (21%), COPD (20%) and asthma (12%). In Tunisia, the percentages of patients with a history of tuberculosis were lower in the other studies. Indeed, Lajnef (29) in his series involving 38 patients, noted a history of tuberculosis in 13.1% of cases, as did Hammami (30) who reported it in 6.4% of cases.This may be related to the endemic situation of tuberculosis in Tunisia, particularly in the central regions including Kairouan, as well as a lower socio-economic level. In other African countries such as Senegal (31) and Congo (32), the antecedent of Tuberculosis was noted in 79% and 50% of cases respectively.On the other hand, in developed countries where the incidence of tuberculosis is lower, this antecedent was reported in only 3.2% of cases in the Pasteur study (21) in Great Britain and 7% in the United States. (33)As infection is an important factor involved in the pathophysiology, post-infection DDB is one of the most commonly identifiable causes in the development of the disease(34). Repeated respiratory infections were the 2nd most common antecedent detected in our series (21%).Our population is similar to that of Kondah (35) in Morocco, who in a retrospective study of 85 cases reported 15% of repeat infections. Ketifi (36) in Algeria reported this in 10% of cases. A recent study carried out at the Abderrahmen Mami Hospital in Tunisia, aimed at establishing the clinical profile of patients with COPD and DDB, noted that the combination of COPD and DDB constitutes a poor prognostic factor with accelerated decline in respiratory function(37).

The identification of DDB in COPD has been defined as a different clinical phenotype of COPD with greater symptomatic severity, more frequent chronic bronchial infection and exacerbations, and a poor prognosis(38). The relationship between asthma and DDB is still a matter of debate. Asthma may be expressed by recurrent pneumonitis and a symptomatology dominated by hypersecretion and bronchial congestion (109).

Recently, in a study of 1680 asthmatic patients, about 3% had radiographic DLB and about 50% of patients with DLB had severe asthma (110). Patients with severe asthma and coexisting DDB represented a distinct group in terms of disease severity, microbiology and asthma phenotype. Chest CT scans and sputum cultures may help to identify these patients. These results may contribute to early recognition and targeted treatment of this group of patients. (111) Indeed, the coexistence of asthma and DDB is associated with an independent increase in the risk of exacerbation despite lower radiological and clinical severity indices.

This may be explained by the inflammation of the asthmatic airways, which could favour the "Cole's circle" responsible for a higher frequency of exacerbations. (39)In this context, studies have shown that asthma when associated with DDB can constitute an independent risk which accelerates the decline in respiratory function. (40) In our series, asthma was found in 12 cases (12%).

2. CLINICAL DATA :

2.1. Functional signs :

DDB should always be suspected in the presence of recurrent respiratory tract infections. The most frequent symptoms are a persistent cough and constant production of thick, tenacious sputum(41). The extent of this chronic bronchorrhoea, which is often increased during episodes of superinfection, has been correlated with the severity of dyspnoea(42).

In our series, bronchorrhoea was reported in 80% of cases. This result is concordant with the data found by Abdmouleh (18) who in his series of 110 patients hospitalized in the pneumology department at the CHU Hédi Chaker in Sfax, reported bronchorrhea in 81% of cases. Similarly, Saidane (43) conducted a retrospective study of 100 patients with DDB and reported bronchorrhea in 95% of cases. Worldwide, the figures are similar. Pappalettera (44), in Italy, reported bronchorrhoea as the most constant and common symptom present in 85% of cases. The group of patients who present with excessive sputum production but without the consistent finding of bacteria in sputum cultures has been described as having "sterile bronchorrhoea". In this group, sputum samples contain neutrophils and necrotic material but have no detectable pathogens. (45)

Dyspnoea was the second most common warning sign reported in our series (61%). A recent study carried out in the United States (46) showed that dyspnoea can occur in 72 of patients. Dyspnoea usually occurs in patients with extensive DDB. It may also be secondary to concomitant disease, such as chronic bronchitis or emphysema.(46) Compared with patients without associated COPD, those with COPD-associated DDB had greater dyspnoea and more impaired lung function.(47)

Haemoptysis occurs in DDB as a result of erosion of neovascular arterioles and is frequently reported, particularly during exacerbations(48). It is reported as blood-stained sputum in most cases, but can be very abundant and life-threatening (49). In our series, it was reported in 34% of cases. This result is consistent with the findings of Louhaichi (50) who conducted a retrospective study in the Ibn Nafis Pneumology Department in Ariana, including 142 patients, and reported haemoptysis in 30.6% of cases. Because of the heterogeneity of DDB, the clinical manifestations and course of the disease are often highly variable. It is therefore important to carefully assess the physical signs in order to establish an aetiological approach and treatment appropriate to the stage of the disease.

2.2. Physical signs :

Clinical signs of bronchial dilatation are not specific. (51) Persistent bronchial rales are most often found on physical examination. They are sometimes associated with sibilants. Their topography and extent reflect the extent of the bronchial lesions. Foci of crackles may indicate alveolar extension of the infection. (52)In our series, crackling rales were reported in 70% of cases and sibilant rales in 25%. These results are consistent with those found in Tunisia, where Hammami (30) reported a predominance of crackling rales with 36.3% followed by sibilant rales in 20% of cases. In Morocco, Afif (53) also reported crackling rales in 43% of cases and sibilants in 32% of patients.

In a study carried out in New Zealand on 56 patients with bronchial dilatation, 52% had digital hippocratism and radiologically more extensive bronchial dilatation (54). Digital hippocratism was reported in 36% of cases in our series. Some series in Tunisia (30) and Morocco (53) reported similar figures of 34% and 48% respectively.These results testify to the delay in consultation and management of patients, the causes of which have been explained in some studies as neglect of symptoms, socio-cultural and economic factors, and difficulty in accessing medical services. (55) In other cases, these percentages were much lower than our 2%.(9)Signs of right heart failure were reported in 16% of patients in our series. cases. Right ventricular dysfunction occurs in chronic lung disease when chronic hypoxaemia and disruption of the pulmonary vascular beds contribute to increased ventricular afterload. Although the exact prevalence is unknown, right ventricular hypertrophy appears to be a frequent complication of chronic lung disease, and is more common in advanced lung disease(56).

III. PARACLINICAL DATA :

1. IMAGING DATA :

If the diagnosis of bronchial dilatation is evoked on the basis of anamnestic and clinical data, imaging allows us to confirm the diagnosis by specifying the morphology of the dilated bronchi, the extent of the DDB lesions and to search for a local or diffuse cause. Chest X-rays, which are sometimes normal at the start of the disease, are not very sensitive (37% to 47%) but are specific (95%). (57)

In our series, areolar images predominated in 55% of cases, bronchial syndrome in 39% and tubal clearing in 8%.Several studies in the literature have reported similar results with a predominance of areolar images. Afif (53) in his study reported areolar images in 47% of cases and tubal clears in 8.9%. Aloui (58) in his series of 35 patients noted a predominance of areolar images in 97% of cases and tubal clearing in 25.7% of cases. In the series by Eastham and colleagues, 66% of cases diagnosed by chest CT would have been missed by chest X-ray alone; chest CT should be performed when the clinical picture is compatible, despite a normal chest X-ray. (59)In a comparative study between standard chest radiography and HR-CT in 84 patients with DDB, VAN DERBRUGGEN-BOGAARTS (60) found that the sensitivity of standard radiography to detect DDB was 87.8% with a specificity of 74.4%. This study also noted that there was a significant correlation between the severity of DDB on CT-HR and the abnormalities found on standard radiography.Thin-section thoracic CT is considered the GOLD STANDARD for the diagnosis of DDB(14). Because of its safety and good sensitivity and specificity (95%) (24), it can be used to recognise the different lesion forms (cylindrical, cystic or varicose), and to assess the number of lobes affected. The main diagnostic criterion for DDB on chest CT is a ratio of bronchus/arter (B/A) greater than 1, giving the classic kitten-ring appearance (61).

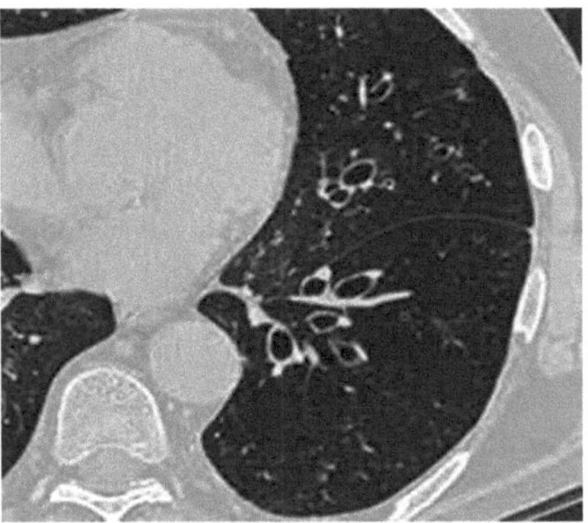

Figure 20: Dilatation of cylindrical bronchi: "kitten ring" appearance.

The CT features of DDB were originally described by Naidich et al, and only minor modifications have been made since (62). The bronchoarterial ratio is the ratio of the diameter of the internal lumen of the bronchus to the adjacent pulmonary artery. Other diagnostic criteria are thickening and irregularity of the bronchial wall, absence of progressive reduction in the calibre of the bronchi in the periphery, and abnormal visibility of bronchial structures in the last subpleural centimetre(63). A hydroaerobic level with dilated bronchi grouped in clusters in cystic DDB. (62)The morphology of DDBs is defined according to Reid's classification based on anatomopathological correlation and bronchography, which divides them into three categories: cylindrical (most frequent), moniliform and cystic(64). In the population studied, cylindrical DDB predominated in 75% of patients, cystic DDB in 52% and varicose DDB in 19%.Our figures are comparable with recent literature. In Tunisia, Saidane (43) in his series of 100 cases of DDB reported similar results with cylindrical DDB in 75% of cases, cystic DDB in 50% of cases and varicose DDB in 10% of cases. Worldwide, Amorim(14) noted in his study 47% cylindrical DDB and 34% cystic DDB with predominant involvement of the lower lobes. In addition to lesion types, CT also enables us to characterise their extent. DDB can be localised or diffuse, and this influences the diagnostic and therapeutic approach. In the case of localised DDB, bronchial fibroscopy is required to assess the airways and look for an obstructive cause. The discovery of diffuse DDB, on the other hand, leads us to look for a systemic cause of the disease. (65) In our series, DDB was diffuse in 67 cases and localised in 33 cases. These results are in line with recent Tunisian studies.

Moussa (66) at the Ibn Nafis Pneumology Department in Ariana reported concordant results with diffuse DDB in 81% of cases. Saidane (43) also noted a diffuse form in 85% of cases. Lesions were unilateral in 22 cases and bilateral in 88.

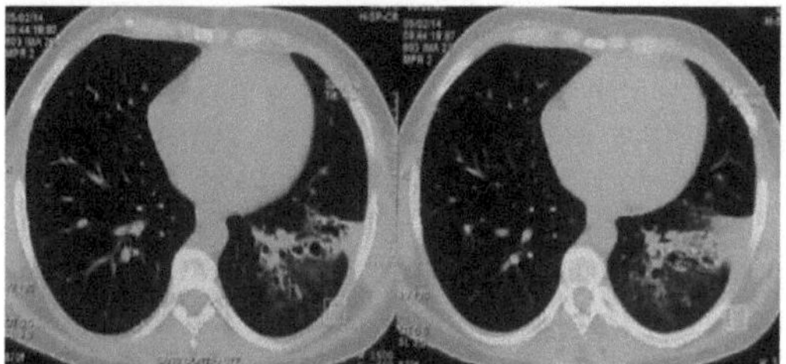

Figure 21: Localized cylindrical bronchial dilatation in the left lower lobe with associated left basal segmental collapse.

2. BIOLOGICAL DATA :

Acute inflammation is an important host defence against bronchial infection; however, if the infection becomes chronic, it can lead to lung damage and disease progression. (67) Stable-phase BMD patients have elevated levels of systemic markers of inflammation; however, this was not dependent on the presence of sputum colonisation.(68) Some markers, in particular neutrophil counts, correlate with disease severity. This finding is consistent with the hypothesis that the level of inflammation determines disease progression. (69)CRP also plays an important role in mediating the extra-pulmonary complications of DDB. It is an important biomarker for the diagnosis and assessment of the frequency and severity of acute exacerbations (AEs) (70). We noted an increase in CRP in 30% of cases in our study. In his series, Hammami reported a correlation between the CRP level on admission and the length of hospitalisation(30).Neutrophils dominate airway inflammation in DDB, driven by high concentrations of neutrophil chemoattractants such as interleukin-8 (CXCL-8) and leukotriene B4. Bacterial colonisation of the respiratory tract is occurs due to impaired mucociliary clearance and failure of phagocytic destruction of neutrophils. (52)In our study, hyperleukocytosis was noted in 18% of cases, with PNN predominating in 10%. A study carried out in Turkie showed that anaemia was associated with signs of and more severe BSI scores. (71) In our study, anaemia was noted in 11% of cases. Platelets are known to contribute to inflammatory processes in addition to their role in thrombosis. A UK study showed that thrombocytosis is associated with disease severity in patients with DDB with higher BSI scores and mortality(72). Thrombocytosis was noted in 7% of cases in our study.

3. MICROBIOLOGICAL DATA :

► Sputum cytobacteriological examination (SCC):

Chronic bacterial infection is common in patients with DDB, and the bronchial inflammation it stimulates has been implicated in the progression of the disease. (73)In this context, ECBC is a key test for monitoring bronchial bacterial colonisation and the effectiveness of antibiotic

therapy. The bacteria most frequently encountered, regardless of aetiology, are Streptococcus Pneumoniae, Haemophilus Influenzae and Pseudomonas Aeruginosa (18). In our series, ECBC was performed in 19 patients, and the germ was isolated in 63% of cases. The following germs were found: Streptococcus pneumoniae in 4 cases (33%), Pseudomonas aeruginosa in 5 cases (42%), Candidas albicans in 2 cases (42%), and Salmonella in 1 case (33%).(17) and Staphylococcus aureus in 1 case (8%).Hammami (30) in his study of 375 patients reported that bacteriological examination made it possible to isolate the germ in 35% of cases, represented essentially by Streptococcus pneumoniae in 28% of cases and pseudomonas aeruginosa in 11%. Infection with Pseudomonas aeruginosa represents a turning point in the evolution of the disease.It is associated with longer hospital stays and higher hospitalisation costs(74).
AP infection is also associated with a high risk of mortality and hospitalisation(75).

- Bronchial fibroscopy :

The discovery of localised SBDs should lead all patients to undergo bronchial fibroscopy as part of the aetiological investigation to look for an obstruction (extrinsic compression or endobronchial obstruction). (76) This examination is also indicated as part of the assessment of haemoptysis (localisation of bleeding) and the search for an endobronchial cause of bleeding, or for microbiological purposes (protected sampling). (18)

Bronchial fibroscopy is also useful in the event of a ventilatory problem (atelectasis), as it can reveal a mucous plug, but above all it can be used to aspirate sticky secretions in order to aerate the lung parenchyma. (77)In our series, 5 of our patients underwent bronchial fibroscopy, which showed a normal appearance in 50% of cases, an inflammatory appearance in 33% and bleeding in 16%. In addition, no endobronchial lesions were found, in particular a bud.stenosis or extrinsic compression.Rabiou (78) in his series of 64 patients operated on for DDB, reported that bronchial fibroscopy performed in 34 cases showed a carcinoid tumour in 1 case, broncholithiasis in 1 case and an intrabronchial foreign body in 1 case.

IV. ETIOLOGICAL ASSESSMENT AND MAIN ETIOLOGIES :

Identifying the aetiology of DDB could influence the management of the disease. and lead to targeted treatments that can improve prognosis. It is It is important to note that, despite extensive research into the aetiology, more than half of all cases of DDB are considered to be idiopathic. (1) In our study, we reported 5% of idiopathic DDB and 39% of undetermined cause (incomplete aetiological work-up).Since the late 1980s, there has been increasing recognition of a population of patients with idiopathic DDB, many of whom are chronically infected with non-tuberculous mycobacteria (NTM). (79) This group of patients consists mainly of postmenopausal, non-smoking women with no known predisposing factors, who present with a chronic cough (80). A high prevalence of cyctic fibrosis transmembrane regulator (CFTR) mutations and signs of ciliary dysfunction have been noted in this population of patients with idiopathic DDB, (81-83) but they do not meet the diagnostic criteria for cystic fibrosis or primary ciliary dyskinesia. These observations suggest that the aetiology of the disease is likely to be multifactorial, in which mucociliary clearance defects may play a key role (84). In our study, post-tuberculosis aetiology accounted for 40%, which is relatively higher than in other studies, given that Tunisia is a country of intermediate endemicity for tuberculosis (85). Abdmouleh (18) in his series of 110 patients hospitalised in the pneumology department of the Hédi Chaker University Hospital in sfax, reported tuberculosis aetiology in 20% of cases. Bejar (19) noted the aetiology of tuberculosis in 25% of cases in his series of 85 patients collected in the pneumology department of the CHU La Rabta in Tunisia.Tuberculosis is an etiology that is essentially present in emerging countries.(86). In France, the people most affected by post-tuberculosis DDB are migrants from North Africa and sub-Saharan Africa. (87)According to the latest figures from the World Health Organisation (WHO), the rate of of tuberculosis decreased by 10%. (86)BBT can cause DDB by various mechanisms: bronchial compression by adenopathy, parenchymal destruction or traction by scar tissue.(88) The DDB are formed austade of sequelae in the area of involvement tuberculosis. The middle lobar bronchus, which is long, small and difficult to drain, is a frequent site of post-tuberculosis DDB (88).Another mechanism for the formation of post-tuberculous DDB is the activation of the immune system via macrophages and lymphocytes: Granulomas. Interactions between the pathogen and the individual's immune response facilitate granulomatous inflammation with tissue damage, e.g. caseation, fibrosis and DDB. (89) Consequently, immunosuppressive and anti-inflammatory drugs such as steroids, new preventive strategies and more effective interventions will be needed to combat these post-tuberculosis sequelae, while assessing their risk-benefit ratios. (90)A major infection in early childhood causes structural damage to the developing lung and leads to bacterial infection, which over time can then lead to DDB. (91) Infections in childhood were for a long time considered to be the almost sole cause of bronchial dilatation (92). In recent decades, thanks to the reduction in pneumopathies occurring in children as a result of the extension of vaccination against measles and whooping cough, its incidence in Western countries has decreased but still represents between 25% and 50% of cases of DDB in adults over the age of 50 (93).In our series we noted 14% of DDB secondary to recurrent infections. These results are consistent with those of Belliraj (94) who reported DLB secondary to recurrent infections in 16% of cases. Some vaccine-preventable diseases, e.g. whooping cough, pneumonia secondary to measles or other infections, can lead to DDB. It is therefore important to ensure that children are up to date with their childhood vaccinations. (95)Cystic fibrosis is a proven cause of bronchial dilatation. Cystic fibrosis is a proven cause of bronchial dilatation, and is increasingly common in adults, given the increased life expectancy of patients with this condition. It is the first etiology to be considered in cases of predominantly upper or moderate bronchial dilatation in young people (15). It is revealed later in incompletely expressed forms, justifying the search for a CFTR gene mutation in the presence of a positive or doubtful sweat test in adults. The The clinical picture is one of DDB, predominantly in the upper lobes, with mucous plugs, mucoid impactions and bronchoceles on imaging, and chronic sinusitis in 100% of cases, as well as male sterility and female hypofertility (91). In a retrospective study of patients with DDB followed at the Pneumology Department of the Hédi Chaker Hospital in Sfax (Tunisia) (78), cystic fibrosis was diagnosed in 2% of cases. In our series, only one case of cystic fibrosis was diagnosed.Finally, it should be noted that the diagnosis of cystic fibrosis is probably underestimated in our patients, due to their lack of resources, which considerably limits investigations in this area. In addition to its vital role in making the diagnosis, thoracic CT in some cases revealed associated signs pointing to a particular aetiology, such as situs inversus, reported in 3 cases in our series, and sequelae of tuberculosis in 21% of cases.The presence of bronchial dilatation predominating at the bases in a child or young adult should raise the possibility of primary ciliary dyskinesia. (39) On CT scan, dilated bronchi predominate in the lower regions and usually have a thickened wall. They are usually associated with mucoid impactions and a budded tree appearance due to a mucociliary clearance defect. (96,97)

Kennedy et al. analysed chest CT scans of 29 adults and 16 children with primary ciliary dyskinesia. The abnormalities found were situs inversus in 38% of cases and heterotaxy in 18%. (98)Louhaichi (50) in his study carried out at the Ibn Nafiss Pneumology Department, Ariana, Tunisia noted ciliary dyskinesia in 4% of cases.In our series, 3 cases of Kartagener's syndrome were detected (3%). The thoracic CT scan may also show evidence of tuberculosis sequelae or active tuberculosis at the origin of the SBDs. Scarring DDB is often associated with fibrous changes in the upper lobes, which can go as far as complete lobar destruction. (99) In active forms, tracheobronchial involvement with the formation of bronchial stenoses may lead to the development of DDB. (99)Bronchial fibroscopy is performed systematically, to determine the inflammatory aspect of the bronchus, anatomical abnormalities, and the abundance and location of purulent secretions. This examination is particularly useful in making an aetiological diagnosis, especially if an airway obstruction (intrinsic or extrinsic) is being investigated. (2) This examination enables essential therapeutic procedures to be carried out, such as the removal of foreign bodies responsible for DDB. (100)Mechanical bronchial obstruction should be systematically sought in the presence of symptomatic localized DLBD. (101)The mechanisms responsible for the onset of localised intracranial bronchial dilatation may be inhalation of a foreign body, which is frequently unrecognised in children who escape surveillance because it occurred several years previously (71,102), or a bronchial tumour, which is essentially benign because malignant tumours develop too quickly to allow bronchial dilatation to develop. These are usually hamartomas, lipomas or carcinoids (103).

Extrinsic obstruction may be due to bronchial compression of lymph node origin, most often developed during primary tuberculosis infection. This compression is responsible for the classic middle lobe syndrome (Brock's syndrome). (104)Bronchogenic cysts of the carina and vascular anomalies compressing the left main bronchus are rare causes of DDB. (105)In the series by FUJIMOTO (106) , bronchial obstruction was found in 14 patients, the cause of which was mainly tuberculosis (9 cases), a foreign body in 3 cases, aspergillosis in one case and a benign tumour in one case.Janah (107) reported the case of a carcinoid tumour discovered in a 32-year-old patient during fibroscopy as part of the aetiological work-up for localised DDB . There have been no reports of foreign bodies, tumours or lymph node compression.in our series.All our patients were tested for BK in the sputum, with positive results in 4 cases. This is consistent with the study by Afif (53) who reported that BK testing was performed in 99.2% of patients. It was positive in 4.5% of cases, resulting in a relapse of parenchymal tuberculosis. Allergic bronchopulmonary aspergillosis (ABPA) may complicate asthma, leading to DDB which is part of the diagnostic criteria for ABPA, or may complicate pre-existing DDB due to another aetiology. Aspergilloma can develop in lung areas containing DDB, while fungal bronchitis can lead to subsequent DDB (108).

The latest ERS recommendations for the management of DDB in adults suggest systematic screening of all patients for allergic bronchopulmonary aspergillosis (ABPA). (109)

In our series, no aspergillary serology was performed. Ketfi (36), in his study of 90 patients hospitalised in the pneumology department at Rouiba in Algeria, reported only one positive aspergillary serology.Faverio (110), in 385 patients, reported ABPA in 4% of cases.DDB can also be caused by a congenital or acquired immune deficiency. Early diagnosis of an immune deficiency can slow the progression of the disease and has an important therapeutic and prognostic impact (111). Most often, the deficiency is related to humoral immunity, but cellular immunity deficiencies may also be involved. Humoral deficiencies are mainly represented by IgA deficiencies, followed by hypogammaglobulinaemia and deficiencies in IgG isotypes. (112,113) Deficiencies in cellular immunity are variably accompanied by deficiencies in antibody production, resulting in an increased incidence of pneumonia, bronchitis and ENT infections, which are a major cause of morbidity and may lead to the formation of diffuse DDB. (114,115)In our study, this test was not routinely performed. One case of variable common immune deficiency CVID has been reported. In the series by Ketfi (36), he reported CVID in 3.3% of cases and acquired immune deficiency in only 1 case. Mark C Pasteur et al (21) found in their series 8% of cases presenting with DDB due to an immune deficiency (humoral in 7% and neutrophil function in 1%).The hypothesis of an association between rheumatoid arthritis (RA) and bronchial dilatation (BDD) has been confirmed by five recent prospective studies (98,116,117) using thin-section CT scans. The prevalence of bronchial dilatation in RA varies from 5% to 30% according to these studies. DDB in RA is most often bilateral, peripheral and associated with bronchiolar involvement. It should be pointed out that RA with symptomatic DDB and obstructive syndrome has a 5-year risk of death which is 5 times higher than that of RA alone(118).In a Tunisian study by ZROUR (96) involving 75 patients with RA, DDB was found in 18.7% of cases. In our series, RA was noted in one patient (1%).The existence of DDB in the context of systemic diseases is a recent development. thanks to the ease with which CT-HR can be performed. In 2016, a retrospective study carried out in Algeria by Ketfi (36) reported that the inventory of systemic diseases associated with DDB was dominated by rheumatoid arthritis (RA) in 50% of cases, Gougerot-Sjögren's syndrome (GSS) in 20% of cases, systemic lupus erythematosus (SLE) in 10% of cases, and haemorrhagic rectocolitis (UC) in 10% of cases.

V. IMPACT ASSESSMENT :

1. RESPIRATORY FUNCTION TESTS :

Considered as a complement to the clinical and radiological examination for DDB, respiratory function tests (RFT) are useful in establishing the impact of the disease both at the time of diagnosis and during therapeutic follow-up (119). Arterial blood gas analysis was performed on admission in 89 patients. It showed hypoxaemia in 27 patients. Ten patients were hypercapnic (PaCO2 2: 45 mm Hg) and 52 had correct blood gases.Our study showed that the median PaO2 was 68 mm Hg. PaCO2 was 40 mm Hg and SaO2 was 90%. According to the series by Moussa (66) arterial blood gas analysis showed: a hypoxaemia in 17% of patients. Hypercapnia was observed in 17% of patients.Spirometry should be performed in a stable state, outside infectious outbreaks. The abnormalities observed reflect the extent of the lesions, their severity and any associated respiratory diseases. (120) Spirometry usually reveals an obstructive ventilatory syndrome with little or no reversibility and a reduction in FEV1. Bronchial hyperresponsiveness may also be present. (121)The association with a restrictive syndrome is frequent, generally due to the presence of atelectasis or non-ventilated territories due to obstructive secretions. (1) In our study, spirometry was performed in 55 patients (55%), showing an obstructive syndrome in 22 patients in the series, a restrictive tendency in 6 cases and a mixed syndrome in 15 patients.This is consistent with the series by Alaoui Yazidi (122) who reported OVD in 36% of cases and Kondah (35) who noted a predominance of obstructive syndrome. A mixed ventilatory disorder was noted in both series, indicating the progressive nature of the disease.In patients with mild-to-moderate steady-state DDB, significant impairment of pulmonary function should raise the alarm about an abnormal chest CT scan or a positive sputum culture for Pseudomonas aeruginosa (123).The 6-minute walk test (TDM6) is a simple exercise test for recording general functional responses of the pulmonary, cardiovascular and muscular systems to assess daily physical activities and quality of life in patients with DDB. (124) Azri (125) in his study of 46 cases of DDB demonstrated that the 6-minute walk test showed an average distance covered of 291.2 m for a mean theoretical value of 523.2 m. Exercise-induced desaturation was noted in 28.3% of cases.A study carried out in Taiwan (126) to assess the correlation between the results of the 6-minute walk test and mortality, showed that patients with a distance-saturation ratio (DSP) of less than 280 m ran a significantly increased risk of death. Hammami (30) in his series noted that 7 patients had a moderate limitation.In our study, CT6 was performed in 10 patients and showed severe limitation in 2 patients and moderate limitation in 5 patients.

2. Cardiovascular check-up :

In extensive and advanced forms of DDB, clinical, electro-cardiographic and possibly echocardiographic signs of chronic pulmonary heart disease should be sought. (127) Pulmonary hypertension (PAH), as a complication of DDB, is associated with increased mortality. (128)In our series we found 3 cases of Chronic Pulmonary Heart Disease (CPC) (3%) and 16 cases of PH (16%). These results are consistent with those of Kondah (35), who reported CPC in 4.2% of cases and PH in 15%. Ketfi (36) reported PH in 10% of cases. Azri (125) reported PH in 28.3% of cases. Gencer (127) studied the impact of DDB on the heart and concluded that ventricular functions are impaired in DDB. Impaired right ventricular function was related to the number of lung lobes involved, arterial oxygen pressure and pulmonary flow acceleration/ejection time. Left ventricular dysfunction was correlated only with right ventricular function (127).

VI. THERAPEUTIC MANAGEMENT :

The aims of treatment for DDB are to prevent exacerbations, reduce symptoms, improve quality of life and halt disease progression. (129) A therapeutic plan should be drawn up for each patient with DDB depending on the degree of severity and symptomatology.

1. MEDICAL TREATMENT:

► Antibiotic therapy :

The use of antibiotics plays a central role in controlling bacterial colonisation. The aim of antibiotics is to treat exacerbations, prevent bacterial infections and eradicate problematic germs. (130)Regular microbiological monitoring of sputum for Pseudomonas colonisation, with subsequent attempts at eradication, reduces the rate of exacerbations. (21,131)

Antibiotic treatment is designed to reduce the bacterial load, as there is a direct relationship between the bacterial load and the extent of airway inflammation and hence the frequency of exacerbations. (132,133)We noted that no long-term antibiotics were prescribed in our series, despite recent studies showing that long-term treatment with macrolides is likely to reduce the frequency of exacerbations and improve quality of life(134).This may be explained by the difficulty patients have in accessing long-term antibiotics.course.A recent review by Laska (135) of the efficacy and safety of inhaled antibiotics for the treatment of adult DDB showed that inhaled antibiotics are well tolerated, reduce the bacterial load and provide a small but statistically significant reduction in the frequency of exacerbations without clinically significant improvement in quality of life in patients with DDB and chronic respiratory tract infections.

According to the latest recommendations of the ERS (109), it has been suggested that adults with DDB with a new isolation of P.aeruginosa should be offered eradication antibiotic therapy. However, eradication antibiotics are not offered to adults with DDB following a new isolation of pathogens other than P. aeruginosa. BTS guidelines recommend that long-term oral antibiotics should be considered for patients with 3 or more exacerbations per year or those colonised with Pseudomonas aeruginosa (136).

The EMBRACE trial (137) showed a benefit in patients with one or more exacerbations per year. In clinical practice, macrolides are most frequently used in patients with three or more exacerbations per year, in patients colonised by Pseudomonas aeruginosa and also in patients with less frequent exacerbations who continue to have significant impairment of quality of life despite standard treatment.

► Anti-inflammatories and immunomodulators :

Bronchial dilatation is due to neutrophil inflammation. The effect of steroids on neutrophils has traditionally been considered minimal; however, there is evidence that steroids induce neutrophil death in vitro (138,139).An overview of literature reviews has shown that regular high-dose inhaled steroids reduce 24-hour sputum volume, reduce inflammatory markers in sputum and improve quality of life.(140) However, they have shown no significant improvement in lung function or frequency of exacerbations. (140)
Elborn (141) has shown that inhaled corticosteroids reduce sputum volume per 24 hours, improve peak expiratory flow and FEV1, and reduce cough score.Welsh (140) found that Steroids used systemically or by inhalation have in most cases shown no significant effect on the decline in lung function and the frequency of exacerbations, and should only be used when indicated because of underlying disease (ABPA, "Asthma-COPD- Overlap-Syndrome"

[ACOS]).A recent study by Toujani (142) showed that the use of inhaled corticosteroids (ICS) in the stable state in patients with DDB is fairly frequent. particularly in patients with co-morbidities. This use could improve symptoms, reduce relapses and the deterioration in respiratory function.

In addition to their antibacterial action, macrolides also have an anti-inflammatory effect, without causing immunosuppression. This effect is based on a reduction in the release of pro-inflammatory cytokines, an increase in the phagocytic function of macrophages, a change in mucus production and a reduction in leucocyte recruitment (143).

There is increasing evidence that prophylactic administration of azithromycin reduces the number of exacerbations and improves quality of life (137); cardiovascular risk does not appear to be increased (137,144).

However, widespread use is not yet recommended, as long-term treatment may be accompanied by increased antibiotic resistance in pneumococcus and non-tuberculous mycobacteria (NTM). (137)

In our series, corticosteroid therapy was prescribed in 88% of our patients, 10 of whom received oral corticosteroids, 18 inhaled corticosteroids and 60 both oral and inhaled corticosteroids. Only one patient received long-term macrolide therapy.

Slim [105] in his series of 68 patients hospitalised in the Pneumology Department, Abderrahmen Mami Hospital, noted that inhaled corticosteroids were prescribed in 7% of cases.

► Bronchodilators :

In a randomised controlled trial in patients with DDB with OVT (but not a primary diagnosis of asthma or COPD), the combination of inhaled formoterol plus budesonide was compared with inhaled budesonide alone (145). The combination group showed improvements in dyspnoea, cough and quality of life (145).In our series, short-acting beta2-mimetics were prescribed in 85 cases (85%), given the comorbidities presented by our group and the heterogeneity of respiratory symptoms. Afif (53) noted that half of their patients were put on bronchodilators of long-acting.According to the latest ERS recommendations, long-acting bronchodilators are not indicated for adult patients with DDB. Bronchodilators are indicated if significant dyspnoea is noted, prior to the use of inhaled mucolytic drugs, and prior to inhaled antibiotics, in order to increase tolerance and optimise lung deposition in diseased areas of the lung (109).Long-term mucolytic therapy (⩾ 3 months) is indicated in adult patients with DDB who have difficulty expectorating with poor quality of life (109).In our series, mucolytics were prescribed in 30% of cases.Bronchial hypersecretion and impaired mucociliary clearance result in an accumulation of mucus in the airways, which facilitates infection and is a source of discomfort (95).Pulmonary rehabilitation is a treatment option for patients with a loss of physical fitness or for those whose daily activity is limited by dyspnoea. The procedure has been shown to improve physical activity and endurance, particularly in patients who also receive targeted respiratory muscle training. (21)

2. SURGICAL TREATMENT :

Despite optimal medical management, some patients will continue to suffer from significant symptoms that affect their quality of life. In these patients, the possibility of a surgical procedure may be evaluated with a view to improving symptoms or slowing their worsening. (106,146)Surgical indications are established in cases of localised and symptomatic DDB. In the various surgical series studied, the main indications for surgery were (8) Recurrent infection (55 to 95% of cases), haemoptysis (3 to 61% of cases), pulmonary empyema or abscess (2 to 11% of cases) and secondary pneumothorax (0 to 3% of cases).In our series, 4 of our patients were referred for surgery. The success rate is reduced despite surgical treatment, particularly in cases with the following characteristics: pseudomonas detected and permanent obstructive pathology. (146) This result suggests that the success rate may be higher if surgery is performed before complications develop.Patients with DDB and advanced lung disease despite adherence to maximal medical management should be considered for referral for transplantation. (147)A recent retrospective study of 34 patients transplanted (33 bipulmonary and 1 monopulmonary) for DDB between 1992 and 2014 found one-year survival of 85% and five-year survival of 73%. (148)The role of recently published indices, the bronchiectasis severity index (BSI) (137) or the FACED score (144) in guiding transplantation requests remains to be defined.

3. ETIOLOGICAL TREATMENT :

In rare cases, a specific therapeutic measure may be appropriate. Immunodeficiency, for example, is an indication for the prescription of intravenous immunoglobulins. Intra-bronchial foreign bodies and bronchial tumours that can be removed also require aetiological treatment.

VII. EVOLUTION AND COMPLICATIONS :

Infectious complications are the most frequent: bacterial colonisation, episodes of bronchial superinfection, pulmonary infection (abscessed or not) or pleural infection. Distant septic localisations (brain abscesses) have become exceptional. Bronchial colonisation by pseudomonas aeroginosa occurs late. (47)In our series, 48 patients (48% of cases) had complications.Severe superinfection was noted in 28 cases, 11 of which were admitted to an intensive care unit.Haemorrhagic complications, which are sometimes revealing, may occur for no apparent reason; these complications represent a threat to the vital prognosis. Haemoptysis is the most frequent complication after bronchopulmonary infection, occurring in over 50% of cases. (18)Jrad (149) in his series of 142 patients reported haemoptysis in 30.6% of cases. These results are comparable to those found by Berny (150) who reported haemoptysis in 38% of cases. All our patients with haemoptysis received medical treatment. Embolisation was not indicated in any patient. A study of 101 patients in Thailand showed that bronchial dilatation accounted for 33% of the causes of massive haemoptysis, followed by tuberculosis in 20% of cases(151). Respiratory failure is most often the result of extensive DDB that has been evolving for many years. It does not differ from other chronic respiratory diseases such as chronic obstructive pulmonary disease. (50)In our series, respiratory failure was noted in 30 cases with recourse to home oxygen and 15 cases required home NIV. These results are in agreement with those noted by Trigui (20) who noted a sewing at home oxygen therapy in 22% of patients.Recent evidence has suggested an increased risk of cardiovascular disease in patients with DDB; it is important to consider other modifiable cardiovascular disease risk factors and their appropriate management. (152,153) Right heart failure may occur late in the course of diffuse DDB (154).Anxiety and depression are common in patients with DDB, with studies showing evidence of depression in 21.1% to 34% and anxiety in 39.8% to 55% of patients. (155,156)

VIII. SEVERITY DIAGNOSIS :

It is important to assess the severity and prognosis of DDB. Due to the complex nature of this condition, severity and prognosis cannot be measured by a single variable, such as FEV1 or the extent of DDB on chest CT. Two tools for predicting the severity and prognosis of DDB have been developed, the BSI and the FACED score. (8,134) The course of DDB is variable and depends mainly on the frequency of exacerbations and P. aeruginosa colonisation. The BSI makes it possible to determine the degree of severity (mild, moderate, severe) of the disease according to various factors (body mass index (BMI), forced expiratory volume in seconds (FEV1), number of hospitalisations, dyspnoea scale, microbiology, number of exacerbations, radiological presentation) and thus to estimate the prognosis. (134,157) In our series, according to the FACED score, the risk of mortality at 5 years was high (12%), moderate (20%) and low (68%). According to the BSI score, the risk of mortality and hospitalisation was high in 71% of cases and moderate in 26%. Saidane (43) in his series of patients, reported that according to the FACED score, the risk of mortality at 5 years was high (26%), moderate (26%) and low (47%). According to the BSI score, the risk of mortality and hospitalisation was high in 67% of cases and moderate in 37%. There was a weak but significant correlation between the two scales: there was a tendency for patients to be classified with a higher BSI compared with the FACED score. This may be explained by the fact that BSI (and not FACED) assesses parameters including BMI, pre-study hospitalisation and exacerbations, chronic colonisation by other micro-organisms and the development of cystic DDB(158).

XRISKOFEXACERBATION :

Despite the frequent use of the term exacerbation in DDB, there is currently no There is no consensual definition of this term in the literature. However, the majority of authors have used the definition of acute change in cough and sputum with the appearance of other symptoms such as dyspnoea, haemoptysis, chest pain and asthenia (159).Exacerbations are associated with an increase in systemic inflammation and an increase in the risk of death. progression of pulmonary lesions. (132) They are frequent and have a major impact on public healthcare expenditure (6). Despite therapeutic advances, almost half of all DDB patients in Europe have at least two exacerbations per year. (134)

Exacerbations are associated with an increase in mortality, a deterioration of respiratory function and poor quality of life(160).The frequency of exacerbations is therefore a prognostic factor and one of the most important aspects of the disease.clinical severity of the disease. Consequently, the majority of clinical trials and therapeutic interventions are aimed at preventing these exacerbations.In this part of our study, we attempted to identify factors predictive of frequent exacerbations (>= 2)(161).In our study, a higher risk of exacerbation was noted in patients with a history of tuberculosis. Clinical signs predictive of exacerbation were dyspnoea, hypoxaemia and respiratory failure at the time of diagnosis. These features are indicative of the severity of the disease at the time of diagnosis.Radiologically, diffuse DDB were predictive of exacerbations.Colonisation with pseudomonas aeroginosa also influenced the number of exacerbations The presence of a TVO was also associated with a higher risk of exacerbation.Recent data have identified the extent of radiographic lesions (>2 lobes), cystic appearance, a moderate to severe BSI score and a history of exacerbations in the last 2 years as predictive factors for exacerbation (129,162), which is a good indicator of the risk of exacerbation.consistent with our results.A study carried out in the United Kingdom showed that colonisation by Pseudomonas Aueroginosa is associated with a more rapid decline in lung function. (116)In a study of 84 patients, Béjar (163) showed that young age, the duration of the disease, the presence of clinical and radiological manifestations, impaired respiratory function and PH could be predictive factors for exacerbations of diffuse DDB. Poor socio-economic conditions such as poverty and undernutrition are also considered predictive factors for exacerbation according to a study carried out in Turkey (164).Particular attention is required for patients with DDB who are overweight, have airway obstruction, have a longer duration of disease, have more severe dyspnoea, have a greater number of lung lobes involved and have one or more comorbidities, in order to correct modifiable risk factors for future exacerbations. (165)Previous hospitalisation, use of proton pump inhibitors, heart failure and BSI or FACED scores were factors associated with the development of exacerbations requiring hospitalisation. Vaccination against pneumococcus was protective. This information may be useful in designing preventive strategies and more intensive follow-up plans. (166)The presence of TVO in patients with DDB is a risk factor of acute exacerbations requiring hospitalisation(162).The number of acute exacerbations is directly related to wall thickness bronchial(163)An increase in PNN inflammation is associated with an increase in the number of exacerbations(164,165).The coexistence of COPD or asthma in patients with DDB has been widely recognised to increase the risk of exacerbations. (167,168) In particular, a meta-analysis of patients with COPD presenting with SBD on CT scan described a marked increase in the risk of exacerbation. (169) In asthmatic patients, the combination of has only been described in severe patients (170,171) in whom the severity of obstruction seems to be associated with the risk of exacerbation, but its predictive value is low. (171)

X. OUTLOOK :

DDB remains a disabling disease with a major socio-economic impact. The best way to manage it is to :

-Preserve the lung's defences by giving up smoking and eliminating other bronchial irritants. (166)

-The treatment of all infectious sites in the teeth and sinuses, which must be an integral part of the treatment process, is essential.to prevent the progression and spread of infections.

-Appropriate management of episodes of lung infection in children, to prevent bronchial dilatation due to childhood infections.

-Annual influenza vaccination. Indirect evidence suggests that this vaccination reduces morbidity, mortality and the cost of care in at-risk populations(167).

-Raising parents' awareness of the benefits of vaccination in preventing respiratory infections: vaccination against measles, whooping cough and tuberculosis in children.

-Early diagnosis of conditions that predispose to the development of PBD, such as ciliary dyskinesia and immune deficiency. Indeed, it has been shown that patients diagnosed late with primary ciliary dyskinesia had a more deteriorated respiratory function due to delayed management of infections and symptoms(168).

In fact, DDB remains a little-known, even mysterious, pathology in newly-diagnosed patients. In this context, a national day could be useful in clarifying the various clinical signs and aetiologies of DDB.

Offer training seminars on this disease, with primary care physicians as the target population, to enable early diagnosis.

CONCLUSION

DDB develops as a result of a recurrent or persistent inflammatory process in the airways, which leads to irreversible changes in the bronchi and is associated with a clinical syndrome characterised by cough, sputum and recurrent respiratory infections. Because of the chronicity of DDB and its complications, this disease is responsible for a high health cost and social handicap.The aim of our work was to describe the epidemiological, clinical, radiological and evolutionary profile of branch dilatations and the factors predictive of exacerbations while referring to the comparative literature. Our study was a retrospective descriptive study of patients hospitalised in the pneumology department of Ibn Al Jazzar Hospital in Kairouan, from January 2010 to September 2020.During the study period, 100 patients were diagnosed with DDB.The average age of the study population was 57.79 years, with extremes ranging from 17 to 90 years. Our population was predominantly female (sex ratio M/F= 0.81) and 69% came from rural areas. The smoking rate was 36.3%, with a male majority of 37%.The pathological history was marked by the predominance of respiratory pathologies. Tuberculosis was predominant in 40% of patients, followed by recurrent respiratory infections in 21% and asthma in 12% of cases. Extra-respiratory conditions were dominated by cardiovascular disease (12%), followed by diabetes (10%).Productive cough was the main presenting sign (80%), followed by dyspnoea (61%). Haemoptysis was noted in 34% of cases, altered general condition in 26% and chest pain in 24%.Physical examination revealed polypnoea in 40 patients (40%) with signs of struggle in 31% (13.7%). Pulmonary auscultation showed a predominance of snoring rales in 51.9% of patients, followed by rales in 2.5% of patients.crepitus in 70% and sibilant rales in 25%. In 36% of patients a digital hippocratism and 16% had signs of right ventricular failure.Radiologically, we noted the presence of the following on the chest X-ray areolar opacities in 55 patients (55%).The diagnosis was confirmed by chest CT in all patients. Cylindrical, cystic and varicose images predominated, with rates of 75%, 52% and 19% respectively. Situs inversus was present in 3% of cases. Lesions were diffuse in 67%, bilateral in 88% and unilateral in 22% of patients.Biologically, hyperleukocytosis was detected in 18% of cases and leukopenia in 2%. CRP was positive in 30% of cases.Microbiological status was recorded using data from ECBC results, which were performed on 19 patients. We isolated the germ in 63% of cases. The germs found were: Streptococcus pneumoniae in 4 cases, Pseudomonas aeruginosa in 5 cases, Candidas albicans in 2 cases and Staphylococcus aureus in 1 case. Direct examination for BK in sputum was positive in 4 patients, i.e. 4% of the population studied.An aetiology was selected in 68 cases, i.e. 68%. We noted a predominance of post-tuberculous DDB in 40 cases, followed by DDB secondary to repeated infections in 14 cases.Post-radiation DDB in 4 cases and kartagener's syndrome in 3 cases. 29 cases.the aetiology remains undetermined. Spirometry was performed in 55 patients (55%), including 22 with obstructive syndrome, 6 with restrictive syndrome and 15 with mixed syndrome.Ten patients (10%) underwent a walking test. Sixty patients (60%) underwent cardiac ultrasound. This led to a diagnosis of chronic pulmonary heart disease (CPC) in 16 patients.In terms of treatment, initial antibiotic therapy was probabilistic in 96 patients.(96%).The drug most commonly used as monotherapy was Amoxicillin-acid The mean duration of antibiotic treatment was 7 days, with extremes ranging from 1 day to 26 days. Respiratory physiotherapy was used in 70 patients (70%).As far as treatments associated with antibiotic therapy were concerned, corticosteroid therapy was the most common.administered IV in 35% of cases. In the stable state, inhaled corticosteroids were indicated in 88% of cases, B2 mimetics in 85% of cases and mucolytics in 30%.Surgical treatment was indicated in 4 patients (4%).The evolution of our patients was marked by the onset of CKD in 30% of cases.Diagnosis of severity was assessed by FACED and BSI scores. According to the FACED score, the risk of mortality at 5 years was high (12%) and moderate (20%). According to the BSI score, the risk of mortality and hospitalisation was high in 71% of cases and moderate in 26%.In our study eight factors were identified as having a significant influence on the number of exacerbations in the last two years, a history of tuberculosis (p=0.002) was associated with a higher risk of exacerbations. There was no significant difference between patients with a history of COPD (p=0.91) and those who smoked (p=0.81).Among the clinical signs, the presence of dyspnoea as a revealing sign (p=0.003) and the presence of hypoxaemia (p=0.003) were associated with a higher number of exacerbations.We also noted that the presence of PH on cardiac ultrasound (p=0.048) and the discovery of respiratory failure (p=0.005) were correlated with more frequent exacerbations. Among the germs found on ECBC, the presence of pseudomonas aeroginosa (p=0.002) was also predictive of exacerbation. On chest CT, diffuse distribution of lesions (p=0.053) was associated with a higher risk of exacerbations.At the end of this study, it should be emphasised that DDB is a real public health problem. The clinical picture is variable, and the aetiologies are multiple, ranging from the presence of a foreign body to the presence of a genetic anomaly. Aetiologies indeterminate remain fairly frequent in our work, given the difficulty of carrying out an exhaustive aetiological work-up due to a lack of resources.Despite advances in treatment, the impact of this condition on patients' quality of life remains remarkable. Optimal management requires not only clear therapeutic objectives (improving the patient's quality of life, avoiding recurrence and treating the corresponding aetiology), but also knowledge of the factors that predict exacerbation.The high percentage of immediately severe forms suggests a delay in consultation and diagnosis. Further studies are needed to investigate the factors influencing these delays.

REFERENCES

1. Bronchial dilatation: a review of 294 cases - ScienceDirect [Internet]. [cited 6 Oct 2021]. Available from: https://www.sciencedirect.com/science/article/abs/pii/S0761842515009109

2. Oumellal J. Surgical treatment of bronchial dilatation in children (about 36 cases) [Internet] [Thesis]. 2010 [cited 6 Oct 2021]. Available from: http://ao.um5.ac.ma/xmlui/handle/123456789/541

3. Etiological diagnosis of bronchial dilatation - ScienceDirect [Internet]. [cited 6 Oct 2021]. Available from: https://www.sciencedirect.com/science/article/abs/pii/S0761841718302165

4. Contarini M, Shoemark A, Rademacher J, Finch S, Gramegna A, Gaffuri M, et al. Why, when and how to investigate primary ciliary dyskinesia in adult patients with bronchiectasis. Multidisciplinary Respiratory Medicine. 2018 Aug 9; 13(1):26.

5. Weycker D, Hansen GL, Seifer FD. Prevalence and incidence of noncystic fibrosis bronchiectasis among US adults in 2013. Chron Respir Dis. nov 14(4):377-84.2017;

6. Living with bronchiectasis [Internet]. Swiss Medical Journal. [cited 6 Oct 2021]. Available from: https://www.revmed.ch/revue-medicale-suisse/2017/revue- medicale-suisse-583/vivre-avec-des-bronchiectasies

7. Reid LMcA. Reduction in Bronchial Subdivision in Bronchiectasis. Thorax. Sept 1950;5(3):233-47.

8. Hill AT, Haworth CS, Aliberti S, Barker A, Blasi F, Boersma W, et al. Pulmonary exacerbation in adults with bronchiectasis: a consensus definition for clinical research. European Respiratory Journal [Internet]. 1 June 2017 [cited 16 Oct 2021];49(6). Available from: https://erj.ersjournals.com/content/49/6/1700051

9. Masson E. Bronchial dilatation: predictive factors of bronchial colonisation [Internet]. EM-Consulte. [cited 8 Oct 2021]. Available from: https://www.em-consulte.com/article/1343158/dilatation-des-bronches -facteurs-predictifs-de-co

10. Iglesias M, Belda J, Baldó X, Gimferrer JM, Catalán M, Rubio M, et al [Bronchial carcinoid tumor: a retrospective analysis of 62 surgically treated cases]. Arch Bronconeumol. May 2004;40(5):218-21.

11. Couderc L-J, Catherinot E, Rivaud E, Guetta L, Mellot F, Cahen P, et al [Are investigations for underlying causes needed for the management of an adult patient with bronchiectasis?]. Rev Pneumol Clin. Sept 2011;67(4):267-74.

12. Amorim A, Bento J, Vaz AP, Gomes I, de Gracia J, Hespanhol V, et al. Bronchiectasis: a retrospective study of clinical and aetiological investigation in a general respiratory department. Rev Port Pneumol (2006). Feb 2015;21(1):5-10.

13. Chassagnon G, Brun A-L, Bennani S, Chergui N, Freche G, Revel M-P. [Bronchiectasis

imaging]. Rev Pneumol Clin. Oct 2018;74(5):299-314.

14. Lonni S, Chalmers JD, Goeminne PC, McDonnell MJ, Dimakou K, De Soyza A, et al. Etiology of Non-Cystic Fibrosis Bronchiectasis in Adults and Its Correlation to Disease Severity. Ann Am Thorac Soc. Dec 2015;12(12):1764-70.

15. Quint JK, Millett ERC, Joshi M, Navaratnam V, Thomas SL, Hurst JR, et al. Changes in the incidence, prevalence and mortality of bronchiectasis in the UK from 2004- 2013: a population based cohort study. Eur Respir J. Jan 2016;47(1):186-93.

16. Abdmouleh K, Feki W, Fekih W, Kallel N, Moussa N, Bahloul N, et al. Radioclinical and aetiological profile of diffuse bronchial dilatation in Tunisia. Revue des Maladies Respiratoires Actualités. Jan 2020;12(1):222-3.

17. Factors associated with impaired lung function in adults with diffuse bronchial dilatation - ScienceDirect [Internet]. [cited 8 Oct 2021]. Available from: https://www.sciencedirect.com/science/article/abs/pii/S0761842516308427

18. Masson E. Current profile of bronchial dilatation [Internet]. EM-Consulte. [cited 8 Oct 2021]. Available from: https://www.em-consulte.com/article/1101318/profil- actuel-des-dilatations-des-bronches

19. Pasteur MC, Helliwell SM, Houghton SJ, Webb SC, Foweraker JE, Coulden RA, et al. An investigation into causative factors in patients with bronchiectasis. Am J Respir Crit Care Med. Oct 2000;162(4 Pt 1):1277-84.

20. Prevalence and incidence of bronchiectasis in Catalonia, Spain: A population-based study - ScienceDirect [Internet]. [cited 8 Oct 2021]. Available from: https://www.sciencedirect.com/science/article/pii/S0954611116302670

21. Grenier P, Maurice F, Musset D, Menu Y, Nahum H. Bronchiectasis: assessment by thin-section CT. Radiology. Oct 1986;161(1):95-9.

22. Currie DC, Cooke JC, Morgan AD, Kerr IH, Delany D, Strickland B, et al. Interpretation of bronchograms and chest radiographs in patients with chronic sputum production. Thorax. Apr 1987;42(4):278-84.

23. Management of bronchial dilatation, what a challenge? A case report of 57 patients - ScienceDirect [Internet]. [cited 8 Oct 2021]. Available from: https://www.sciencedirect.com/science/article/abs/pii/S1877120319316210

24. Boucher RC. Relationship of airway epithelial ion transport to chronic bronchitis. Proc Am Thorac Soc. 2004;1(1):66-70.

25. Risk factors for bronchiectasis in patients with chronic obstructive pulmonary disease: a systematic review and meta-analysis - PubMed [Internet]. [cited 8 Oct 2021]. Available from: https://pubmed.ncbi.nlm.nih.gov/33886788/

26. Mull ES, Shell R, Adler B, Holtzlander M. Bronchiectasis associated with electronic

cigarette use: A case series. Pediatr Pulmonol. Dec 2020;55(12):3443-9.

27. Lajnef H. Diffuse bronchiectasis in adults, radio-clinical approach and etiological profile. 2009.

28. Hammami khawla. clinical profile and therapeutic management of bronchial dilatation. 2018.

29. Indications and outcomes of pulmonary emphysema bulla resection surgery [Internet]. [cited 8 Oct 2021]. Available from: https://www.panafrican-med-journal.com/content/article/31/48/full/

30. Profil épidémiologique de dilatation des bronches au service de pneumologie du CHU de Brazzaville - PDF Free Download [Internet]. coek.info. [cited 8 Oct 2021]. Available from: https://coek.info/pdf-profil-epidemiologique-de-dilatation-des- bronches-au-service-de-pneumologie-du-c.html

31. Jordan TS, Spencer EM, Davies P. Tuberculosis, bronchiectasis and chronic airflow obstruction. Respirology. May 2010;15(4):623-8.

32. Hsieh M-H, Fang Y-F, Chen G-Y, Chung F-T, Liu Y-C, Wu C-H, et al. The role of the high-sensitivity C-reactive protein in patients with stable non-cystic fibrosis bronchiectasis. Pulm Med. 2013;2013:795140.

33. Radio-clinical and etiological aspects of bronchiectasis in the pneumology department of Hôpital Militaire A [Internet]. [cited 8 Oct 2021]. Available from: http://webcache.googleusercontent.com/search?q=cache:M31XkpayP6EJ:wd.fmpm.uca.ma/biblio/theses/annee-htm/FT/2018/these72- 18.pdf+&cd=1&hl=en&ct=clnk&gl=tn

34. Ketfi A, Ihadadene D, Hachi S, Jaafar M, Chabati O, Gharnaout M. Etiological profile of bronchial dilatation. Journal of Respiratory Diseases. 1 Jan 2017;34:A250.

35. Habouria C, Bachouch I, Belloumi N, Harizi C, Chermiti F, Fenniche S. Bronchial dilatations associated with chronic obstructive pulmonary disease: clinical and evolutionary profile. Pan Afr Med J. 18 Nov 2020;37:249.

36. Martinez-Garcia MA, Miravitlles M. Bronchiectasis in COPD patients: more than a comorbidity? Int J Chron Obstruct Pulmon Dis. May 11, 2017;12:1401-11.

37. Honoré I, Burgel P-R. Primary ciliary dyskinesia in adults. Rev Mal Respir. Feb 2016;33(2):165-89.

38. Keistinen T, Säynäjäkangas O, Tuuponen T, Kivelä SL. Bronchiectasis: an orphan disease with a poorly-understood prognosis. Eur Respir J. Dec 1997;10(12):2784-7.

39. Masson E. Bronchial dilatation [Internet]. EM-Consulte. [cited 8 Oct 2021]. Available from: https://www.em-consulte.com/article/26132/dilatations-des- bronchial tubes

40. Ellis D. Present outlook in bronchiectasis: clinical and social study and review of factors

influencing-prognosis. 1986;

41. Masson E. Radico-clinical, therapeutic and evolutionary profile of patients with DDB: about 100 cases [Internet]. EM-Consulte. [cited 8 Oct 2021]. Available from: https://www.em-consulte.com/article/1343160/profil-radio-clinique- therapeutique-et-evolutif-de

42. Pappalettera M, Aliberti S, Castellotti P, Ruvolo L, Giunta V, Blasi F. Bronchiectasis: an update. Clin Respir J. Jul 2009;3(3):126-34.

43. Smith DJ. Phenotyping bronchiectasis: is it all about sputum and infection? Eur Respir J. Apr 2016;47(4):1037-9.

44. Bronchiectasis: Practice Essentials, Background, Pathophysiology [Internet]. [cited 8 Oct 2021]. Available from: https://emedicine.medscape.com/article/296961- overview

45. King PT, Holdsworth SR, Farmer M, Freezer N, Villanueva E, Holmes PW. Phenotypes of adult bronchiectasis: onset of productive cough in childhood and adulthood. COPD. Apr 2009;6(2):130-6.

46. Bronchiectasis - an overview | ScienceDirect Topics [Internet]. [cited 8 Oct 2021]. Available from sur:https://www.sciencedirect.com/topics/medicine-and-dentistry/bronchiectasis

47. Bird K, Memon J. Bronchiectasis. In: StatPearls [Internet]. Treasure Island (FL): StatPearls Publishing; 2021 [cited 8 Oct 2021]. Available from: http://www.ncbi.nlm.nih.gov/books/NBK430810/

48. Louhaichi S, Smadhi H, Kamoun H, Rouiss H, Ben Abdelghaffar H, Greb D, et al. Clinical, aetiological and evolutionary aspects of patients followed for bronchial dilatation. Journal of Respiratory Diseases. Jan 1, 2019;36:A145.

49. SmithMP.Diagnosis and management of bronchiectasis. CMAJ. 19 June 2017;189(24):E828-35.

50. Bird K, Memon J. Bronchiectasis. In: StatPearls [Internet]. Treasure Island (FL): StatPearls Publishing; 2021 [cited 8 Oct 2021]. Available from: http://www.ncbi.nlm.nih.gov/books/NBK430810/

51. Afif M. Dilatations des bronches (à propos de 247 cas) These Med Casablanca n 274. 2006.

52. Edwards EA, Metcalfe R, Milne DG, Thompson J, Byrnes CA. Retrospective review of children presenting with noncystic fibrosis bronchiectasis: HRCT features and clinical relationships. Pediatr Pulmonol. August 2003;36(2):87-93.

53. Aetiologies of bronchial dilatation in children: about 44 cases - EM consults [Internet]. [cited 8 Oct 2021]. Available from: https://www.em- consulte.com/article/1101332/les-etiologies-des-dilatations-de-bronches-chez-l-

54. Kolb TM, Hassoun PM. Right Ventricular Dysfunction in Chronic Lung Disease. Cardiol Clin. May 2012;30(2):243-56.

55. Bronchiectasis : American Journal of Roentgenology : Vol. 193, No. 3 (AJR) [Internet]. [cited 8 Oct 2021]. Available from: https://www.ajronline.org/doi/full/10.2214/AJR.09.3053?mobileUi=0

56. Clinical profile of bronchial dilatations hospitalised at the Pneumology Department of the Med VI University Hospital in Marrakech from January 2005 to December 2010 [Internet]. [cited 8 Oct 2021]. Available from: https://123dok.net/document/6zkw1pzx-clinique-dilatations-bronches-hospitalises-pneumologie-marrakech-janvier-dcembre.html

57. Eastham KM, Fall AJ, Mitchell L, Spencer DA. The need to redefine non-cystic fibrosis bronchiectasis in childhood. Thorax. Apr 2004;59(4):324-7.

58. van der Bruggen-Bogaarts BA, van der Bruggen HM, van Waes PF, Lammers JW. Assessment of bronchiectasis: comparison of HRCT and spiral volumetric CT. J Comput Assist Tomogr. Feb 1996;20(1):15-9.

59. Cantin L, Bankier AA, Eisenberg RL. Bronchiectasis. American Journal of Roentgenology. Sep 1, 2009;193(3):W158-71.

60. Naidich DP, McCauley DI, Khouri NF, Stitik FP, Siegelman SS. Computed tomography of bronchiectasis. J Comput Assist Tomogr. June 1982;6(3):437-44.

61. Grenier P-A, Beigelman-Aubry C, Brillet P-Y, Lenoir S. [Bronchial diseases: CT imaging features]. J Radiol. Nov 2009;90(11 Pt 2):1801-18.

62. Reiff DB, Wells AU, Carr DH, Cole PJ, Hansell DM. CT findings in bronchiectasis: limited value in distinguishing between idiopathic and specific types. AJR Am J Roentgenol. August 1995;165(2):261-7.

63. Livnat G, Bentur L. Non-cystic fibrosis bronchiectasis: review and recent advances. F1000 Med Rep. 26 August 2009;1:67.

64. Journal of Respiratory Diseases [Internet]. [cited 8 Oct 2021]. Available from: https://www.rev-mal-respir.com/article/1343163/profil-radio-clinique-et- etiologique-des-dilatatio

65. Robb CT, Regan KH, Dorward DA, Rossi AG. Key mechanisms governing resolution of lung inflammation. Semin Immunopathol. Jul 2016;38(4):425-48.

66. Menéndez R, Méndez R, Amara-Elori I, Reyes S, Montull B, Feced L, et al. Systemic Inflammation during and after Bronchiectasis Exacerbations: Impact of Pseudomonas aeruginosa. J Clin Med. August 13, 2020;9(8):2631.

67. Wilson CB, Jones PW, O'Leary CJ, Hansell DM, Dowling RB, Cole PJ, et al. Systemic markers of inflammation in stable bronchiectasis. Eur Respir J. Oct 1998;12(4):820-4.

68. Liang Y, Chang C, Zhu H, Shen N, He B, Yao W. Correlation between decrease of CRP and resolution of airway inflammatory response, improvement of health status, and clinical outcomes during severe acute exacerbation of chronic obstructive pulmonary disease. Intern Emerg Med. Sep 2015;10(6):685-91.

69. Niksarlioglu EYO, Uysal MA, Yigitba□ B, K1l1ç L, Çamsar1 G. Impact of Anemia On Clinically Stable Adult Non-cystic Fibrosis Bronchiectasis. European Respiratory Journal [Internet]. 15 Sep 2018 [cited 8 Oct 2021];52(suppl 62). Available from: https://erj.ersjournals.com/content/52/suppl_62/PA788

70. Renton D, Hill J, Abo-Leyeh H, Finch S, Crichton M, Fardon T, et al. Thrombocytosis is associated with disease severity and outcomes in stable bronchiectasis. European Respiratory Journal [Internet]. 2015 Sep 1 [cited 2021 Oct 16];46(suppl 59). Available from: https://erj.ersjournals.com/content/46/suppl_59/OA469

71. O'Donnell AE. Medical managementN of bronchiectasis. J Thorac Dis. Oct 2018;10(Suppl 28):S3428-35.
Cost of Hospitalizations due to Exacerbation in Patients with Non-Cystic Fibrosis Bronchiectasis - Abstract - Respiration 2018, Vol. 96, No. 5 - Karger Publishers [Internet]. [cited 16 Oct 2021]. Available from: https://www.karger.com/Article/Abstract/489935

72. A Comprehensive Analysis of the Impact of Pseudomonas aeruginosa Colonization on Prognosis in Adult Bronchiectasis - PubMed [Internet]. [cited 16 Oct 2021]. Available from: https://pubmed.ncbi.nlm.nih.gov/26356317/

73. Bronchial syndrome - EM consults [Internet]. [cited 8 Oct 2021]. Available from: https://www.em-consulte.com/article/1061025/syndrome-bronchique

74. Chang AB, Redding GJ. Bronchiectasis and Chronic Suppurative Lung Disease. Kendig's Disorders of the Respiratory Tract in Children. 2019;439-459.e6.

75. Rabiou S, Issoufou I, Ammor FZ, Harmouchi H, Belliraj L, Lakranbi M, et al. Surgical results in 64 patients operated for bronchial dilatation. Journal of Clinical Pulmonology. Sep 1, 2017;73(4):199-205.

76. Prince DS, Peterson DD, Steiner RM, Gottlieb JE, Scott R, Israel HL, et al. Infection with Mycobacterium avium complex in patients without predisposing conditions. N Engl J Med. 28 Sep 1989;321(13):863-8.

77. Reich JM, Johnson RE. Mycobacterium avium complex pulmonary disease presenting as an isolated lingular or middle lobe pattern. The Lady Windermere syndrome. Chest. June 1992;101(6):1605-9.

78. Fowler CJ, Olivier KN, Leung JM, Smith CC, Huth AG, Root H, et al. Abnormal nasal nitric oxide production, ciliary beat frequency, and Toll-like receptor response in pulmonary nontuberculous mycobacterial disease epithelium. Am J Respir Crit Care Med. June 15, 2013;187(12):1374-81.

79. Ziedalski TM, Kao PN, Henig NR, Jacobs SS, Ruoss SJ. Prospective analysis of cystic fibrosis transmembrane regulator mutations in adults with bronchiectasis or pulmonary

nontuberculous mycobacterial infection. Chest. Oct 2006;130(4):995-1002.

80. Kim RD, Greenberg DE, Ehrmantraut ME, Guide SV, Ding L, Shea Y, et al. Pulmonary nontuberculous mycobacterial disease: prospective study of a distinct preexisting syndrome. Am J Respir Crit Care Med. 15 Nov 2008;178(10):1066-74.

81. Luisetti M, Pignatti PF. Genetics of idiopathic disseminated bronchiectasis. Semin Respir Crit Care Med. Apr 2003;24(2):179-84.

82. Global tuberculosis report 2020 [Internet]. [cited 8 Oct 2021]. Available from: https://www.who.int/publications/i/item/9789240013131

83. Global tuberculosis report 2020 [Internet]. [cited 8 Oct 2021]. Available from: https://www.who.int/publications-detail-redirect/9789240013131

84. Etiological investigation of adult bronchiectasis - EM consults [Internet]. [cited 8 Oct 2021]. Available from: https://www.em- consulte.com/article/93865/enquete-etiologique-devant-des-bronchectasies-de-l

85. Non-CF bronchiectasis: does knowing the aetiology lead to changes in management? | European Respiratory Society [Internet]. [cited 8 Oct 2021]. Available from: https://erj.ersjournals.com/content/26/1/8

86. Tuberculosis as a Cause of Upper Lobe Bronchiectasis [Internet]. [cited 8 Oct 2021]. Available from: https://www.ncbi.nlm.nih.gov/pmc/articles/PMC1520760/

87. Akram A. Tuberculosis-Induced Bronchiectasis Complicated by Recurrent Respiratory Tract Infections and Renal Amyloidosis: A Classic Revisited. Cureus [Internet]. 23 nov 2020 [quoted 8 Oct 2021];12(11).Available from:

https://www.cureus.com/articles/45499-tuberculosis-induced-bronchiectasis- complicated-by-recurrent-respiratory-tract-infections-and-renal-amyloidosis-a- classic-reviewed

88. King PT. The pathophysiology of bronchiectasis. Int J Chron Obstruct Pulmon Dis. 2009;4:411-9.

89. Bronchiectasis: a re-emerging disease [Internet]. Swiss Medical Journal. [cited 8 Oct2021].Available on:https://www.revmed.ch/revue-medicale- suisse/2007/revue-medicale-suisse-99/bronchiectasies-a-pathology-that-re-emerges

90. Management of Chronic Bronchial Sepsis Due to Bronchiectasis: Clinical Pulmonary Medicine [Internet]. [cited 8 Oct 2021]. Available from: https://journals.lww.com/clinpulm/abstract/1994/11000/management_of_chronic_ bronchial_sepsis_due_to.2.aspx

91. Masson E. Clinical and aetiological manifestations of bronchial dilatation in children according to sex [Internet]. EM-Consulte. [cited 8 Oct 2021]. Available from: https://www.em-consulte.com/rmr/article/1266982

92. Immunisation Handbook 2020 [Internet]. Ministry of Health NZ. [cited 8 Oct 2021]. Available from: https://www.health.govt.nz/publication/immunisation-handbook- 2020

93. A longitudinal study characterising a large adult primary ciliary dyskinesia population | European Respiratory Society [Internet]. [cited 8 Oct 2021]. Available from: https://erj.ersjournals.com/content/48/2/441

94. Frija-Masson J, Bassinet L, Honoré I, Dufeu N, Housset B, Coste A, et al. Clinical characteristics, functional respiratory decline and follow-up in adult patients with primary ciliary dyskinesia. Thorax. feb 2017;72(2):154-60.

95. Kennedy MP, Noone PG, Leigh MW, Zariwala MA, Minnix SL, Knowles MR, et al. High-resolution CT of patients with primary ciliary dyskinesia. AJR Am J Roentgenol. May 2007;188(5):1232-8.

96. Beigelman C, Sellami D, Brauner M. CT of parenchymal and bronchial tuberculosis. Eur Radiol. 2000;10(5):699-709.

97. Kechna H, Ouzzad O, Aissaoui Y, Nadour K, Zaini R. Extraction of a tracheobronchial foreign body using a uretheroscope. Pan Afr Med J. 28 Jan 2015;20:74.

98. Surgery for localized bronchial dilatation [Internet]. [cited 8 Oct 2021]. Availablesur: http://webcache.googleusercontent.com/search?q=cache:CeqV8HzWiGsJ:wd.fmp m.uca.ma/biblio/theses/annee-htm/FT/2015/these31- 15.pdf+&cd=1&hl=en&ct=clnk&gl=tn

99. Davies G, Wells AU, Doffman S, Watanabe S, Wilson R. The effect of Pseudomonas aeruginosa on pulmonary function in patients with bronchiectasis. Eur Respir J. Nov 2006;28(5):974-9.

100. Benign bronchopulmonary tumours - EM consults [Internet]. [cited 8 Oct 2021]. Available from: https://www.em-consulte.com/article/31085/tumeurs- benign-bronchopulmonary

101. A case of middle lobe syndrome - EM consults [Internet]. [cited 8 Oct 2021]. Available from: https://www.em-consulte.com/article/93984/un-cas-de-syndrome- middle-lobe-syndrome

102. Masson E. P228 - An exceptional observation of trans mural bronchogenic cyst of the carina [Internet]. EM-Consulte. [cited 8 Oct 2021]. Available from: https://www.em-consulte.com/article/259564

103. Fujimoto T, Hillejan L, Stamatis G. Current strategy for surgical management of bronchiectasis. Ann Thorac Surg. Nov 2001;72(5):1711-5.

104. Localized bronchial dilatation revealing a carcinoid tumor [Internet]. [cited 8 Oct 2021]. Available from: https://www.panafrican-med- journal.com/content/article/24/278/full/

105. Bronchiectasis and Aspergillus: How are they linked? | Medical Mycology | Oxford Academic [Internet]. [cited 8 Oct 2021]. Available from:

https://academic.oup.com/mmy/article/55/1/69/2408143?login=true

106. European Respiratory Society guidelines for the management of adult bronchiectasis [Internet]. [cited 8 Oct 2021]. Available from: https://erj.ersjournals.com/content/50/3/1700629

107. ABPA screening in bronchiectasis: is there a grey zone? | European Respiratory Society [Internet]. [cited 8 Oct 2021]. Available from: https://erj.ersjournals.com/content/52/suppl_62/PA2677

108. Bronchiectasis - Pulmonary disorders [Internet]. Professional edition of the MSD. [cited 8 Oct 2021]. Available at: https://www.msdmanuals.com/fr/professional/troubles-pulmonary/bronchiectasis-and-at%C3%A9lectasis/bronchiectasis

109. Masson E. Primary immune deficiencies [Internet]. EM-Consulte. [cited 8 Oct 2021]. Available from: https://www.em-consulte.com/article/846/deficits- immunodeficiency-primitive

110. De Gracia J, Rodrigo MJ, Morell F, Vendrell M, Miravitlles M, Cruz MJ, et al. IgG subclass deficiencies associated with bronchiectasis. Am J Respir Crit Care Med. Feb 1996;153(2):650-5.

111. Bard M, Couderc LJ, Saimot AG, Scherrer A, Frachon I, Seigneur F, et al. Accelerated obstructive pulmonary disease in HIV-infected patients with bronchiectasis. Eur Respir J. March 1998;11(3):771-5.

112. Verghese A, al-Samman M, Nabhan D, Naylor AD, Rivera M. Bacterial bronchitis and bronchiectasis in human immunodeficiency virus infection. Arch Intern Med. 26 Sep 1994;154(18):2086-91.

113. Honoré I, Burgel P-R. Primary ciliary dyskinesia in adults. Rev Mal Respir. Feb 2016;33(2):165-89.

114. Masson E. Enquête étiologique devant des bronchectasies de l'adulte [Internet]. EM-Consulte. [cited 8 Oct 2021]. Available from: https://www.em-consulte.com/article/93865/enquete-etiologique-devant-des-bronchectasies-de-l

115. Yunt ZX, Solomon JJ. Lung Disease in Rheumatoid Arthritis. Rheum Dis Clin North Am. May 2015;41(2):225-36.

116. van Zeller M, Mota PC, Amorim A, Viana P, Martins P, Gaspar L, et al. Pulmonary rehabilitation in patients with bronchiectasis: pulmonary function, arterial blood gases, and the 6-minute walk test. J Cardiopulm Rehabil Prev. Oct 2012;32(5):278-83.

117. Lamb K, Theodore D, Bhutta BS. Spirometry. In: StatPearls [Internet]. Treasure Island (FL): StatPearls Publishing; 2021 [cited 8 Oct 2021]. Available from: http://www.ncbi.nlm.nih.gov/books/NBK560526/

118. Lopes AJ, Camilo GB, de Menezes SLS, Guimarães FS. Impact of Different Etiologies

of Bronchiectasis on the Pulmonary Function Tests. Clin Med Res. March 2015;13(1):12-9.

119. Alaoui Y. Clinical profile of bronchial dilatations hospitalised in the pneumology department of the Med VI University Hospital in Marrakech from January 2005 to December 2010 N
106. 2012.

120. Evans SA, Turner SM, Bosch BJ, Hardy CC, Woodhead MA. Lung function in bronchiectasis: the influence of Pseudomonas aeruginosa. Eur Respir J. August 1996;9(8):1601-4.

121. ATS Committee on Proficiency Standards for Clinical Pulmonary Function Laboratories. ATS statement: guidelines for the six-minute walk test. Am J Respir Crit Care Med. 1 Jul 2002;166(1):111-7.

122. Revue des Maladies Respiratoires Actualités - Vol 13 - n° 1 - EM consult [Internet]. [cited 8 Oct 2021]. Available from: https://www.em- consulte.com/revue/RMRA/13/1/table-of-matters/

123. Hsieh M-H, Fang Y-F, Chung F-T, Lee C-S, Chang Y-C, Liu Y-Z, et al. Distance-saturation product of the 6-minute walk test predicts mortality of patients with non-cystic fibrosis bronchiectasis. J Thorac Dis. Sep 2017;9(9):3168-76.

124. Gencer M, Ceylan E, Yilmaz R, Gur M. Impact of bronchiectasis on right and left ventricular functions. Respir Med. Nov 2006;100(11):1933-43.

125. Wang L, Jiang S, Shi J, Gong S, Zhao Q, Jiang R, et al. Clinical characteristics of pulmonary hypertension in bronchiectasis. Front Med. Sep 2016;10(3):336-44.

126. King PT, Holdsworth SR, Freezer NJ, Villanueva E, Holmes PW. Characterisation of the onset and presenting clinical features of adult bronchiectasis. Respir Med. Dec 2006;100(12):2183-9.

127. CISMeF. CISMeF [Internet]. Rouen University Hospital; [cited 8 Oct 2021]. Available from: https://www.cismef.org/page/dilatation-des-bronches

128. White L, Mirrani G, Grover M, Rollason J, Malin A, Suntharalingam J. Outcomes of Pseudomonas eradication therapy in patients with non-cystic fibrosis bronchiectasis. Respir Med. March 2012;106(3):356-60.

129. Chalmers JD, Smith MP, McHugh BJ, Doherty C, Govan JR, Hill AT. Short- and long-term antibiotic treatment reduces airway and systemic inflammation in non-cystic fibrosis bronchiectasis. Am J Respir Crit Care Med. 1 Oct 2012;186(7):657-65.

130. Serisier DJ, Bilton D, De Soyza A, Thompson PJ, Kolbe J, Greville HW, et al. Inhaled, dual release liposomal ciprofloxacin in non-cystic fibrosis bronchiectasis (ORBIT-2): a randomised, double-blind, placebo-controlled trial. Thorax. Sep 2013;68(9):812-7.

131. Chalmers JD, Goeminne P, Aliberti S, McDonnell MJ, Lonni S, Davidson J, et al. The bronchiectasis severity index. An international derivation and validation study. Am J Respir Crit Care Med. March 1, 2014;189(5):576-85.

132. Laska IF, Crichton ML, Shoemark A, Chalmers JD. The efficacy and safety of inhaled antibiotics for the treatment of bronchiectasis in adults: a systematic review and meta-analysis. Lancet Respir Med. Oct 2019;7(10):855-69.

133. Hill AT, Sullivan AL, Chalmers JD, De Soyza A, Elborn SJ, Floto AR, et al. British Thoracic Society Guideline for bronchiectasis in adults. Thorax. Jan 2019;74(Suppl 1):1-69.

134. Wong C, Jayaram L, Karalus N, Eaton T, Tong C, Hockey H, et al. Azithromycin for prevention of exacerbations in non-cystic fibrosis bronchiectasis (EMBRACE): a randomised, double-blind, placebo-controlled trial. Lancet. 18 August 2012;380(9842):660-7.

135. Schleimer RP. Effects of glucocorticosteroids on inflammatory cells relevant to their therapeutic applications in asthma. Am Rev Respir Dis. Feb 1990;141(2 Pt 2):S59-69.

136. Dexamethasone-induced suppression of apoptosis in human neutrophils requires continuous stimulation of new protein synthesis - Cox - 1997 - Journal of Leukocyte Biology - Wiley Online Library [Internet]. [cited 8 Oct 2021]. Available from: https://jlb.onlinelibrary.wiley.com/doi/abs/10.1002/jlb.61.2.224

137. Interventions for bronchiectasis: an overview of Cochrane systematic reviews [Internet]. [cited 8 Oct 2021]. Available at: https://www.cochrane.org/CD010337/AIRWAYS_interventions-bronchiectasis- overview-cochrane-systematic-reviews

138. Elborn JS, Johnston B, Allen F, Clarke J, McGarry J, Varghese G. Inhaled steroids in patients with bronchiectasis. Respir Med. March 1992;86(2):121-4.

139. Prescribing inhaled corticosteroids in bronchiectasis - EM consults [Internet]. [cited 8 Oct 2021]. Available from: https://www.em- consulte.com/article/1419645/prescribing-inhaled-corticosteroids-in-bronchiectasis - EM consulte [Internet].

140. Kanoh S, Rubin BK. Mechanisms of action and clinical application of macrolides as immunomodulatory medications. Clin Microbiol Rev. July 2010;23(3):590-615.

141. Serisier DJ, Martin ML, McGuckin MA, Lourie R, Chen AC, Brain B, et al. Effect of long-term, low-dose erythromycin on pulmonary exacerbations among patients with non-cystic fibrosis bronchiectasis: the BLESS randomized controlled trial. JAMA. March 27, 2013;309(12):1260-7.

142. Martínez-García MÁ, Soler-Cataluña JJ, Catalán-Serra P, Román-Sánchez P, Tordera MP. Clinical efficacy and safety of budesonide-formoterol in non-cystic fibrosis bronchiectasis. Chest. Feb 2012;141(2):461-8.

143. Ashour M, Al-Kattan KM, Jain SK, Al-Majed S, Al-Kassimi F, Mobaireek A, et al. Surgery for unilateral bronchiectasis: results and prognostic factors. Tuber Lung Dis. Apr

1996;77(2):168-72.

144. Martínez-García MÁ, de Gracia J, Vendrell Relat M, Girón R-M, Máiz Carro L, de la Rosa Carrillo D, et al. Multidimensional approach to non-cystic fibrosis bronchiectasis: the FACED score. Eur Respir J. May 2014;43(5):1357-67.

145. Diagnosis and management of bronchiectasis | CMAJ [Internet]. [cited 8 Oct 2021]. Available from: https://www.cmaj.ca/content/189/24/E828

146. Weill D, Benden C, Corris PA, Dark JH, Davis RD, Keshavjee S, et al. A consensus document for the selection of lung transplant candidates: 2014--an update from the Pulmonary Transplantation Council of the International Society for Heart and Lung Transplantation. J Heart Lung Transplant. Jan 2015;34(1):1-15.

147. Therapeutic and evolutionary aspects of patients treated for bronchial dilatation - ScienceDirect [Internet].[cited8 Oct2021].Available at: https://www.sciencedirect.com/science/article/abs/pii/S1877120320305796

148. Bronchial dilatations: about 294 cases - EM consults [Internet]. [cited 8 Oct 2021]. Available from: https://www.em-consulte.com/article/1023232/les- bronchial-dilation%C2%A0-about-294%C2%A0cases

149. Reechaipichitkul W, Latong S. Etiology and treatment outcomes of massive hemoptysis. Southeast Asian J Trop Med Public Health. March 2005;36(2):474-80.

150. Navaratnam V, Millett ERC, Hurst JR, Thomas SL, Smeeth L, Hubbard RB, et al. Bronchiectasis and the risk of cardiovascular disease: a population-based study. Thorax. Feb 2017;72(2):161-6.

151. Evans IES, Bedi P, Quinn TM, Hill AT. Bronchiectasis Severity Is an Independent Risk Factor for Vascular Disease in a Bronchiectasis Cohort. Chest. Feb 2017;151(2):383-8.

152. Bopaka RG, Janah H, Jabri H, Bemba ELP, Okemba-Okombi FH, Khattabi WE, et al. Kartagener syndrome revealed in adulthood. Annale des Sciences de la Santé [Internet]. 20 Jan 2017 [cited 8 Oct 2021];16(2). Available from: https://www.annalesumng.org/index.php/ssa/article/view/250

153. Girón Moreno RM, Fernandes Vasconcelos G, Cisneros C, Gómez-Punter RM, Segrelles Calvo G, Ancochea J. Presence of anxiety and depression in patients with bronchiectasis unrelated to cystic fibrosis. Arch Bronconeumol. Oct 2013;49(10):415-20.

154. Ôzgün Niksarlioglu EY, Ôzkan G, Günlüoglu G, Uysal MA, Gül S, Kilic L, et al. Factors related to depression and anxiety in adults with bronchiectasis. Neuropsychiatr Dis Treat. 2016;12:3005-10.

155. Ellis HC, Cowman S, Fernandes M, Wilson R, Loebinger MR. Predicting mortality in bronchiectasis using bronchiectasis severity index and FACED scores: a 19-year cohort study. Eur Respir J. Feb 2016;47(2):482-9.

156. Costa JC, Machado JN, Ferreira C, Gama J, Rodrigues C. The Bronchiectasis Severity Index and FACED score for assessment of the severity of bronchiectasis. Pulmonology. 3 Jan 2018;S2173-5115(17)30154-9.

157. Polverino E, Dimakou K, Hurst J, Martinez-Garcia MA, Miravitlles M, Paggiaro P, et al. The overlap between bronchiectasis and chronic airways diseases: state of the art and future directions. European Respiratory Journal [Internet]. 1 Jan 2018 [cited 16 Oct 2021]; Available sur: https://erj.ersjournals.com/content/early/2018/07/12/13993003.00328-2018

158. Clinical phenotypes in adult patients with bronchiectasis | European Respiratory Society [Internet]. [cited 16 Oct 2021]. Available from: https://erj.ersjournals.com/content/47/4/1113

159. Chang AB, Bilton D. Exacerbations in cystic fibrosis: 4--Non-cystic fibrosis bronchiectasis. Thorax. March 2008;63(3):269-76.

160. Khalid M, Saleemi S, Zeitouni M, Al Dammas S, Khaliq MR. Effect of obstructive airway disease in patients with non-cystic fibrosis bronchiectasis. Ann Saudi Med. August 2004;24(4):284-7.

161. Ooi GC, Khong PL, Chan-Yeung M, Ho JCM, Chan PKS, Lee JCK, et al. High-resolution CT quantification of bronchiectasis: clinical and functional correlation. Radiology. Dec 2002;225(3):663-72.

162. Wilson CB, Jones PW, O'Leary CJ, Hansell DM, Dowling RB, Cole PJ, et al. Systemic markers of inflammation in stable bronchiectasis. European Respiratory Journal. 1 Oct 1998;12(4):820-4.

163. Tsang KW, Chan K, Ho P, Zheng L, Ooi GC, Ho JC, et al. Sputum elastase in steady-state bronchiectasis. Chest. Feb 2000;117(2):420-6.

164. Shin MS, Ho KJ. Bronchiectasis in patients with alpha 1-antitrypsin deficiency. A rare occurrence? Chest. Nov 1993;104(5):1384-6.

165. Sehatzadeh S. Influenza and Pneumococcal Vaccinations for Patients With Chronic Obstructive Pulmonary Disease (COPD). Ont Health Technol Assess Ser. March 1, 2012;12(3):1-64.

166. Ellerman A, Bisgaard H. Longitudinal study of lung function in a cohort of primary ciliary dyskinesia. Eur Respir J. Oct 1997;10(10):2376-9.

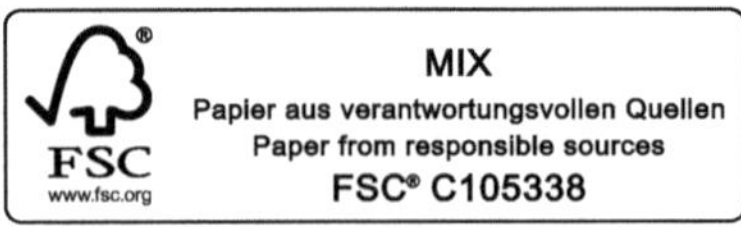

Printed by Books on Demand GmbH, Norderstedt / Germany